Premenstrual Syndrome: Current Findings and Future Directions

The
PROGRESS IN PSYCHIATRY
Series

David Spiegel, M.D., Series Editor

SPRING 1985

The Borderline:
Current Empirical Research
Edited by Thomas H. McGlashan, M.D.

Premenstrual Syndrome:
Current Findings and Future Directions
*Edited by Howard J. Osofsky, M.D., Ph.D.,
and Susan J. Blumenthal, M.D.*

Treatment of Affective Disorders in the Elderly
Edited by Charles A. Shamoian, M.D., Ph.D.

Premenstrual Syndrome: Current Findings and Future Directions

Edited by
Howard J. Osofsky, M.D., Ph.D.
Susan J. Blumenthal, M.D.

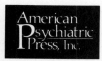

1400 K Street, N.W., Suite 505
Washington, DC 20005

Copyright © 1985 American Psychiatric Association
ALL RIGHTS RESERVED
Manufactured in the United States of America

Library of Congress Cataloging in Publication Data

Premenstrual syndrome.

(The Progress in psychiatry series)
Based on a symposium held during the 137th Annual Meeting of the American Psychiatric Association, held in Los Angeles, May 8, 1984.
Includes bibliographies.
1. Premenstrual syndrome—Congresses. I. Osofsky, Howard J. 1935–   . II. Blumenthal, Susan J. 1952–   . III. American Psychiatric Association. Meeting (137th: 1984: Los Angeles, Calif.) IV. Series. [DNLM: 1. Premenstrual Tension—congresses. WP 560 P9237 1984]
RG165.P74   1985   618.1′72   85-6100
ISBN 0-88048-071-8

Contents

Contributors

Sheryle W. Alagna, Ph.D.
Assistant Professor of Medical Psychology, Uniformed Services University
of Health Sciences

Susan J. Blumenthal, M.D.
Head, Suicide Research Unit, Center for Studies of Affective Disorders,
National Institute of Mental Health

Paula Clayton, M.D.
Professor and Head, Department of Psychiatry, University of Minnesota
Medical School

Jean Endicott, Ph.D.
Chief, Department of Research Assessment and Training,
New York State Psychiatric Institute

Ira D. Glick, M.D.
Professor of Psychiatry, Department of Psychiatry; and Associate Medical
Director, Payne Whitney Psychiatric Clinic, The New York
Hospital–Cornell Medical Center

Gay N. Grover, M.S.N.
Staff Nurse, National Institutes of Health

Uriel Halbreich, M.D.
Associate Professor of Psychiatry, Albert Einstein College of Medicine of
Yeshiva University

Jean A. Hamilton, M.D.
Head, Biology of Depression Research Unit, Center for Studies of
Affective Disorders (Visiting Scientist from the University of
Chicago), National Institute of Mental Health; and Director,
Institute for Research on Women's Health

M. Christine Hoban, M.S.W.
Social Worker, National Institutes of Health

William Keppel, M.D.
Staff Psychiatrist, The Menninger Foundation

John Nee, Ph.D.
Biostatistician, Department of Research Assessment and Training, New York State Psychiatric Institute

Howard J. Osofsky, M.D., Ph.D.
Psychiatry Discipline Chief, The Menninger Foundation

Barbara L. Parry, M.D.
Senior Staff Fellow, Clinical Psychobiology Branch, National Institute of Mental Health

Robert M. Post, M.D.
Chief, Clinical Psychobiology Branch, National Institute of Mental Health

Norman E. Rosenthal, M.D.
Chief, Outpatient Services, Clinical Psychobiology Branch, National Institute of Mental Health

Peter Roy-Byrne, M.D.
Staff Psychiatrist, National Institute of Mental Health

David R. Rubinow, M.D.
Chief, Psychiatry Consultation-Liaison; and Chief, Unit on Peptide Studies, National Institute of Mental Health

Sybil Schacht, M.S.W.
Research Scientist, Department of Research Assessment and Training, New York State Psychiatric Institute

Kathey Sharpe, M.A.
Psychology Department, George Washington University; and Psychology Fellow, Washington, D.C. General Hospital

Thomas A. Wehr, M.D.
Chief, Clinical Psychobiology Branch, National Institute of Mental Health

Introduction to the Progress in Psychiatry Series

The *Progress in Psychiatry* Series is designed to capture in print the excitement that comes from assembling a diverse group of experts from various locations to examine in detail the newest information about a developing aspect of psychiatry. This series emerged as a collaboration between the American Psychiatric Association's Scientific Program Committee and the American Psychiatric Press, Inc. Great interest was generated by a number of the symposia presented each year at the APA Annual Meeting, and we realized that much of the information presented there, carefully assembled by people who are deeply immersed in a given area, would unfortunately not appear together in print. The symposia sessions at the Annual Meetings provide an unusual opportunity for experts who otherwise might not meet on the same platform to share their diverse viewpoints for a period of three hours. Some new themes are repeatedly reinforced and gain credence, while in other instances disagreements emerge, enabling the audience and now the reader to reach informed decisions about new directions in the field. The *Progress in Psychiatry* Series allows us to publish and capture some of the best of the symposia and thus provide an in-depth treatment of specific areas which might not otherwise be presented in broader review formats.

The symposia are selected on the basis of review by the Symposium Subcommittee of the Scientific Program Committee. From the approximately 80 symposia a year selected for presentation at the Annual Meeting, we choose approximately 10 percent which are deemed to be of especially high quality and to have interest to readers as well as meeting participants. After review by the American Psychiatric Press, we invite the authors to submit their papers as manuscripts for publication. We make every effort to expedite the publishing process so that books in the *Progress in Psychiatry* Series will be available as close as possible to the time of presentation at the Annual Meeting.

We believe the *Progress in Psychiatry* Series will provide you with an opportunity to review timely new information in specific fields of interest as they are developing. We hope you find that the excitement of the presentations is captured in the written word and that this book proves to be informative and enjoyable reading.

David Spiegel, M.D.
Series Editor
Progress in Psychiatry Series

Foreword

After reading and thinking about the chapters in this book, I am reminded of two important works from modern psychiatry. In *The Vital Balance*, Karl Menninger said, "There are many ways to organize miscellaneous data and classification is one of the basic devices for bringing order out of chaos, both in the universe and in our own thinking." Later he said, "A new classification can be very fruitful if it helps put old observations in a new light and generates new questions for research." This book attempts to do exactly what Karl Menninger advocates: to extract knowledge from a large body of opinion and information in order to shed new light on clinically important syndromes and generate new questions. In doing so the authors have begun to establish diagnostic validity. Robins and Guze (1970) described five phases in the development of a valid classification. The first phase is clinical description, which is the main thrust of what is attempted in the chapters that follow. The second phase is laboratory studies. These have been carefully reviewed in a number of the chapters. As accurately pointed out, the laboratory studies that are currently available in general provide few clearly reliable or reproducible results. The third phase is the delimitation from other disorders. A number of the chapters have attempted both to delimit the entities and relate them when appropriate to other clinical disorders. As expected, such delimitation and integration are more complex and difficult to achieve than simple clinical description. Phases four and five are follow-up studies and family studies. These obviously must be done after two of the first three phases, clinical description and delimitation, are accomplished.

These chapters are helpful to anyone wanting to understand the knowledge base for premenstrual syndrome(s). They are critical, where appropriate, of previous work, whether it be the definition of the syndrome(s), methods developed to study it, treatment protocols, or outcomes. Unlike previous reports, these have no obvious bias in the reporting. The chapters give needed information on baseline values of physiological, psychological, and cognitive assessments during phases of the menstrual cycle and report on new data relevant to clinical conceptualization, evaluation, and treatment.

The book reports on studies that can be regarded as hypothesis generating. It lays the groundwork for hypothesis testing. When the reader completes this monograph, he or she will know where the field has been, where it is now, and where it should be in 10 years.

Paula Clayton, M.D.

REFERENCES

Menninger K, Mayman M, Pruyser P: The Vital Balance: The Life Process in Mental Health and Illness. New York, Penguin Books, 1979

Robins E, Guze SB: Establishment of diagnostic validity in psychiatric illness: its application to schizophrenia. Am J Psychiatry 126:107–111, 1970

Introduction

Although premenstrual tension was first described in 1931, it has been primarily in recent years that the medical profession has given growing recognition to the importance of symptoms that appear linked to the menstrual cycle. Also, and perhaps related in part to the feminist movement and to women's insistence on better care for themselves, more women have openly described symptoms to their physicians, and physicians in turn have become more cognizant that these problems deserve attention. Adding further impetus to the interest in this area have been the publications by the British physician Katharina Dalton, who has advocated progesterone therapy for the premenstrual syndrome. In recent years, both in England and in the United States, there have been court cases in which the premenstrual syndrome was claimed as a defense for acts of violence. It seems likely that the incidence of such cases is likely to grow. Under any circumstances, the area is an important one and deserves careful attention.

Investigators have used different names to describe the symptom complexes that women experience: premenstrual tension, premenstrual syndrome, premenstrual symptoms, premenstrual changes. Because of the variety and varying intensity of symptoms along with the clustering of certain symptoms, a number of investigators prefer to use the term *premenstrual syndromes*. Estimates indicate that many women of childbearing age have some premenstrual symptoms and that 3 percent to 15 percent have severe symptoms. Physical symptoms include swelling, weight gain, feeling bloated or fat, pain in the breasts, acne, symptoms of an allergic nature, headaches, clumsiness or awkwardness, or difficulties with concentration or memory. Psychological symptoms include feelings of anger, irritability, nervousness, food cravings, decreased (or increased) energy levels and sexual desire, feelings of unreality, or depression, including suicidal feelings. When emotional symptoms are severe, they are most commonly linked to disturbances of mood or affect. However, there are suggestions that a variety of disorders, for example, bulimia, worsen premenstrually, and some psychotic episodes appear linked to a menstrual cycle.

In this book, we are attempting to present some of the most current information in this complex area, as well as likely directions for future developments. In the first chapter, Drs. Endicott and Halbreich and their colleagues address research approaches to the identification and classification of premenstrual symptoms and links between premenstrual affective changes and the lifetime history of major affective disorders. In the next chapter, Drs. Halbreich and Endicott review the endocrinology of the menstrual cycle, biological hypotheses for the etiology of premenstrual changes, limitations in the data currently available concerning hypotheses, and possible directions for future research. Dr. Rubinow and his colleagues deal with methodological issues that arise in the effort to gain both a research and a clinical understanding of menstrually related mood disorders. They consider the importance of a careful definition of the symptoms and the need for prospective assessment of symptoms. They further consider questions concerning possible relationships between menstrually related mood changes and formal psychiatric disorders, including whether psychiatric syndromes and premenstrual syndromes are concurrent but separate disorders, whether premenstrual symptoms can mimic major psychiatric disorders, whether there is a premenstrual entrainment of major psychiatric disorders, whether there can be a premenstrual exacerbation of psychiatric disorders, whether premenstrual symptoms can be a sensitizing experience influencing the course or development of major psychiatric syndromes, and whether there are etiological commonalities between premenstrual mood syndromes and major psychiatric syndromes that may allow for better understanding of both models.

Chapters 4, 5, and 6 involve a fuller exploration of clinical approaches for evaluation, understanding, and treatment of menstrually related symptoms. Drs. Osofsky and Keppel deal with psychiatric and gynecological components of evaluation and treatment, focusing primarily on physical symptoms and mild to moderate emotional symptoms. Prospective evaluations are detailed, and the efficacy of various treatment approaches are considered, including exercise, modification of diet, vitamin supplementation, progesterone and progestagen compounds, diuretics, bromocriptine, and antiprostaglandins. Dr. Glick deals with more severe symptoms, including the rationale for and treatment of affective, schizophrenic, and borderline personality disorders. In his presentation, he discusses the use of psychotropic medications, as well as the question of the place of hormonal treatment in these conditions. Dr. Hamilton and her colleagues describe the links between cognition and symptoms related to the menstrual cycle, including questions of change in cognitive performance and possible biological substrates to cognitive symptoms. On the basis of the available data and their own experience, the authors of these three chapters discuss the possible efficacy of individual psychotherapy, family therapy, and cognitive therapy in selected patients.

In the final chapter, Dr. Parry and her colleagues review some of the methodological problems that create difficulties in gaining a better understanding of symptoms related to the menstrual cycle and their possible links to psychiatric disorders. They then discuss some of the important issues that are involved in generating hypotheses and some of the links and similarities between specific psychiatric disorders and symptoms related to the menstrual cycle, links that hold the possibility of determining meaningful future research directions.

We recognize that we remain at an early stage of knowledge in our understanding of an important area and that the tasks confronting us are difficult ones. However, in spite of the considerable limitations that exist in the data, important information is available that can be of help to us in our conceptualizations and in our evaluation and treatment strategies. We hope that the information presented in this monograph will help in providing greater clarity about current conceptualizations in the area. We also hope that in coming years additional methodologically sound information will be gathered that will contribute to further advances in our thinking and approaches to clinical care.

Howard J. Osofsky, M.D., Ph.D.
Susan J. Blumenthal, M.D.

Chapter 1

Affective Disorder and Premenstrual Depression

Jean Endicott, Ph.D.
Uriel Halbreich, M.D.
Sybil Schacht, M.S.W.
John Nee, Ph.D.

Chapter 1

Affective Disorder and Premenstrual Depression

M any clinicians and investigators are interested in premenstrual changes of a depressive or dysphoric nature. This is in part because women sometimes seek treatment for such changes. In addition, many who have been involved in the treatment or follow-up of depressed women have observed premenstrual exacerbations of symptoms or premenstrual episodes of dysphoria in otherwise euthymic women.

Some women develop premenstrual changes that resemble a full depressive syndrome when viewed cross-sectionally. They have dysphoric mood or a loss of interest and pleasure, and they have changes in four or more of the commonly associated depressive symptoms involving such factors as sleep, appetite, energy level, and concentration. The depressive syndrome seen premenstrually does not tend to have prominent "endogenous/melancholic" features, but rather tends to be characterized by such features as labile mood, hypersomnia, anxiety-agitation, irritability, or a feeling of an inability to cope.

The depressive syndrome seen premenstrually thus resembles that seen in outpatients who seek treatment for chronic depression or episodes of major depression rather than that seen in the majority of hospitalized depressed patients. The level of severity of the depressive syndrome and the social impairment associated with it vary considerably. For most women it is relatively mild and may not be readily apparent to others. On the other hand, some women have such severe changes that they are unable to work, unable to function effectively as parents, or are at risk for suicide (Janowsky et al. 1969; Abramowitz et al. 1982; Pallis and Holding 1976; Tonks et al. 1968).

This work was supported in part by the New York State Department of Mental Hygiene, the Albert Einstein College of Medicine, grants MH36186 and MHCRC 30906 from the National Institute of Mental Health, and the Ritten Foundation.

FREQUENCY OF PREMENSTRUAL DEPRESSIVE SYNDROME

How frequent are premenstrual depressive changes? The obvious answer is "it depends." It depends on how they are measured, among which groups of women, the level of severity required, and a number of other yet unidentified factors. The data reported in this paper are limited to those from studies that have used reports made by the women themselves of specific types of premenstrual change which met specified syndromal criteria. Although the criteria vary somewhat among the studies, for the most part they are similar to the DSM-III criteria for a major depressive syndrome on a cross-sectional basis.

None of the sets of criteria for premenstrual depressive changes required a specified duration. Some women report changes that occur only one day prior to and a couple of days into the menstrual cycle (the "paramenstrual" period), while others report that they can detect changes in mood beginning just after ovulation. There is some tendency for women with dysphoric premenstrual changes to have a longer duration of physical, mood, and behavioral changes than women who have physical changes only or who feel better premenstrually.

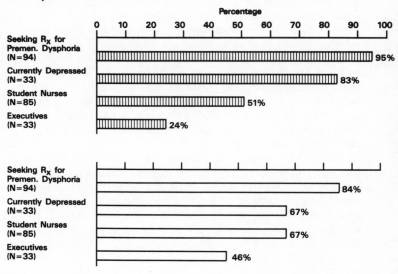

Figure 1. Percentages of Women in Various Subpopulations Who Had Premenstrual Full Depressive Syndrome *(Top)* or Premenstrual Water-Retention Syndrome *(Bottom)*

Figure 1 illustrates the wide variability in reported rates of specific premenstrual changes among various groups of women. These women all completed the Premenstrual Assessment Form (PAF) (Halbreich et al. 1982). The percentage who met the PAF typological category criteria of full depressive syndrome are noted at the top of Figure 1. The women may or may not have also had social impairment. The PAF criteria are such that a very mild depressive syndrome would be noted as long as there were a sufficient number of associated features (Halbreich and Endicott 1982).

The group of women reporting the lowest frequency were lawyers and business women who were major executives or partners in large New York firms. The women with the highest frequencies of reported premenstrual depression were those who were seeking treatment for their premenstrual problems and women with chronic depression seeking treatment in a depression clinic. Figure 1 indicates that the differences in frequency of a water-retention syndrome (e.g., feel bloated, shoes and rings too tight) are not as great. The greater specificity of the depressive syndrome is shown although the water retention and depressive changes are relatively highly correlated among women (in that few women have depressive changes without the physical changes often referred to as "signs of water retention").

ASSOCIATION WITH A LIFETIME DIAGNOSIS OF MAJOR DEPRESSIVE DISORDER

Predicting Premenstrual Depression from Lifetime Diagnosis

One of the earliest studies that used specified criteria for both a lifetime diagnosis of major depressive episode and a premenstrual depressive syndrome was that of Kashiwagi et al. (1976). They noted that women attending a headache clinic who had a lifetime diagnosis of major depressive disorder had a greater likelihood of having a premenstrual affective syndrome (65 percent) than did women who were judged to have "other mental disorder" (14 percent).

The association between a lifetime diagnosis of depressive disorder and a PAF premenstrual depressive syndrome is shown in Figure 2. One hundred ten women diagnosed as having had a "nonpremenstrual" major depressive disorder by Research Diagnostic Criteria (RDC) (Spitzer et al. 1977) had a much higher rate of premenstrual depressive syndrome (57 percent) than did women diagnosed as having never been mentally ill (14 percent). In contrast, the differences in physical changes suggestive of water retention were not as great. (The sources of the women and the procedures used are de-

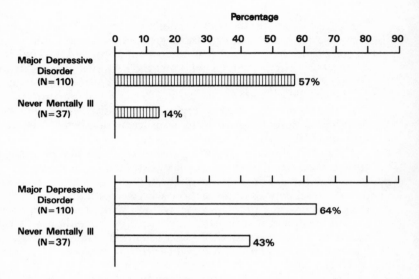

Figure 2. Relationship of Premenstrual Full Depressive Syndrome *(Top)* and Premenstrual Water-Retention Syndrome *(Bottom)* to Lifetime Diagnosis

scribed in greater detail in an article by Halbreich and Endicott [in press].)

Association of Lifetime Diagnosis with Dimensional Measures of Premenstrual Change

Another way of looking at the association of the lifetime diagnosis of major depressive disorder and premenstrual changes is the use of dimensional composite scale scores rather than typological categories. Figure 3 contrasts PAF dimensional scale scores for two groups of women who had responded to a notice seeking subjects to participate in studies of physical condition, mood, and behavior along the menstrual cycle. None of the women met criteria for a current mental disorder. They were categorized on the basis of the RDC into those who had ever met criteria for a nonpremenstrual major depressive disorder, those who had met criteria for some other nonaffective mental disorder, and those who had never been mentally ill. The two extreme groups are contrasted in Figure 3. As was the case with the typological categories, the largest differences between the two groups are on the scales measuring mood and behavior rather than those measuring physical complaints such as edema, feeling of being

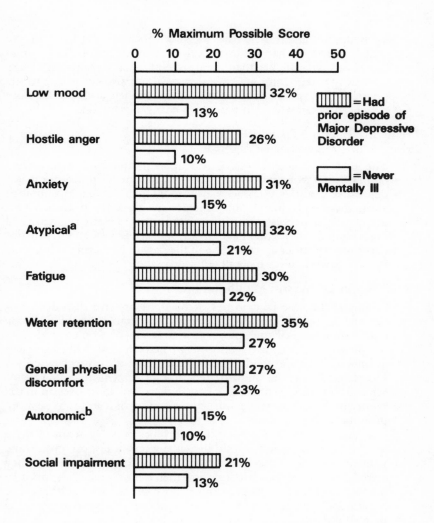

Figure 3. Average Scores on Premenstrual Affect Form Scales for Women Who Had a Prior Episode of Major Depressive Disorder and Women Who Were Never Mentally Ill

[a]Atypical includes hypersomnia, overeating, mood swings, and other depressive features often referred to as atypical.

[b]Autonomic includes features such as rapid heartbeat, sweating, and other changes in the autonomic nervous system.

bloated, joint and muscle pain, rapid heartbeat, or sweating. Figure 3 also illustrates that the disturbances in mood and behavior tend to be somewhat higher than the degree of social impairment. There is no way of knowing whether the social impairment is due to the physical discomfort or the emotional disturbance, and it is therefore measured separately from reports of changes in mood.

Predicting Lifetime Diagnosis from Presence of Premenstrual Diagnosis

The analyses noted above focused upon the rates of premenstrual depression in women with and without a lifetime diagnosis for major depressive disorder. Another way of looking at the relationship is to assess the rates of lifetime major depressive disorder in women with premenstrual depression. Most of the women with premenstrual depression in our studies have already met criteria for an RDC major depressive disorder at some time in the past (84 percent), while only 9 percent were never mentally ill.

Variability in Depressive Manifestations

Just as is the case in episodes of major depressive disorder or in chronic depressive disorders, there is considerable variability in the manifestations. For example, within a group of women with premenstrual full depressive syndrome, 35 percent described themselves as hypersomnic and tending to overeat, while 29 percent described themselves as anxious and agitated, and 42 percent described themselves as hostile or irritable. Of course there was some overlap in the "subtypes," but there is a tendency for one set of features to be more prominent than another.

In addition to the variation in syndromes between women, there are different syndromes within the same woman. For example, some women describe themselves as having had a few days in which they were hypersomnic and lethargic and then a brief period just prior to menses in which they had insomnia and some agitation. Others note a period of feeling better and having more energy followed by a period of depression (Halbreich et al. 1982).

Prognostic Significance of Premenstrual Depressive Syndrome

Two studies are focused upon the prognostic significance of premenstrual depression. Wetzel and his colleagues (1975) evaluated students when they entered college and divided them into a group with premenstrual affective syndrome and a group without a premenstrual affective syndrome. During the ensuing four-year follow-up, 18 percent of those with a premenstrual affective syndrome were diagnosed as developing at least one episode of major affective disorder. Ten percent of those without a premenstrual affective syndrome were so diagnosed. In a somewhat similar study, Schuckit and his colleagues (1975) noted that 7 percent of college students with premenstrual emotional syndrome developed a depressive syndrome during the next 12 months while none of those without the premenstrual emotional syndrome developed a depressive disorder. These two studies suggest that association between retrospective accounts leading to an association between a lifetime diagnosis of major depressive disorder and premenstrual depression are not artifacts of the data-collection procedures but rather a reflection of the increased risk for either condition given the presence of the other condition. Additional prognostic studies of high-risk populations are warranted.

DISCUSSION

The findings presented here as well as observations made by clinicians indicate that there is a high degree of association between premenstrual depressive changes and a lifetime diagnosis of a major depressive disorder. Given that this is the case, what are the implications for research investigators and clinicians?

The clear implication for research investigators is that studies of the relationship between mental disorder and premenstrual changes should focus on specific subtypes of both conditions. Failure to do so in the past probably accounts for some of the inconsistencies in findings. Efforts to find correlates of premenstrual changes, be they biological or social, should take into account subtypes of premenstrual changes as well as the lifetime diagnoses of the subjects. Attention should also be paid to the way in which the sample is recruited.

Given the many changes in mood and behavior and physical as well as biological changes along the menstrual cycle, investigators should always record the phase of the cycle in which a study is being conducted (relative to ovulation or onset of menses). Whenever possible, an investigator should study female subjects in the same phase of the cycle, taking into account that there is less variability in mood and behavior in the week after the cessation of menses than there is in the week prior to menses or the week of ovulation. Furthermore, if an investigator has knowledge of a lifetime diagnosis, it may help predict premenstrual changes in mood and behavior, or at least alert him or her to the likelihood of such changes.

Clinicians particularly need to be alert to the possibility of menstrual cycle-related changes in mood and behavior and physical condition. Many women being treated with medication for chronic depression or anxiety will continue to show some premenstrual changes either in the form of a breakthrough of symptoms or a change in symptoms. These may mistakenly be considered by the clinician to be evidence of side effects of medication, failure of the treatment, or an impending relapse. An awareness of the phase of the cycle may prevent the clinician from acting hastily in changing the medication or, on the other hand, may lead to a planned increase in medication during the latter phases of the menstrual cycle.

Awareness of phases of the menstrual cycle in female patients may also lead clinicians to recognize the periodicity of acting-out behavior, "borderline features," dissatisfaction with therapy, or dissatisfaction with a boyfriend or a job. Such awareness may aid in planning ahead for likely negative behaviors (such as suicide attempts) or in urging the patient to delay making important decisions (such as deciding to quit a job) until after menses have begun.

Increased information regarding the pathophysiology of premenstrual depression may lead to a better understanding of the pathophysiology of similar changes which occur at times other than during the premenstrual period and which occur in men as well as in women. To the degree that premenstrual depressive syndromes can serve as models for similar depressive syndromes that occur at other times, there should be mutual contributions from studies of depressed outpatients and studies of premenstrual dysphoria. Obviously, investigators and clinicians in the two areas should remain aware of the work of those conducting studies in the other area.

REFERENCES

Abramowitz ES, Baker AH, Freischer SP: Onset of depressive psychiatric crises and the menstrual cycle. Am J Psychiatry 139:475–478, 1982

Halbreich U, Endicott J: Classification of the premenstrual cycle, in Behavior and the Menstrual Cycle. Edited by Friedman R. New York, Marcel Dekker, 1982, pp. 245–265

Halbreich U, Endicott J: Methodological issues in studies of premenstrual changes. Psychoneuroendocrinology (in press)

Halbreich U, Endicott J: The relationship of dysphoric premenstrual changes to depressive disorders. J Acta Psychiatr Scand (in press)

Halbreich U, Endicott J, Nee J: The diversity of premenstrual changes as reflected in the premenstrual evaluation form. Acta Psychiatr Scand 65:46–65, 1982

Janowsky DS, Gorney R, Castelnuevo-Tedesco P, et al: Premenstrual-menstrual increases in psychiatric admission rates. Am J Obstet Gynecol 103:189–191, 1969

Kashiwagi T, McClure JN Jr, Wetzel RD: Premenstrual affective syndrome and psychiatric disorder. Dis Nerv Sys 37:116–119, 1976

Pallis D, Holding I: The menstrual cycle and suicidal intent. J Biosoc Sci 8:27–33, 1976

Schuckit MA, Daly V, Herman G, et al: Premenstrual symptoms and depression in a university population. Dis Nerv Sys 39:516–517, 1975

Spitzer RL, Endicott J, Robins R: Research Diagnostic Criteria: rationale and reliability. Arch Gen Psychiatry 35:773–82, 1978

Tonks CM, Rack PH, Rose MJ: Attempted suicide and the menstrual cycle. J Psychosom Res 11:319–323, 1968

Wetzel RD, Reich T, McClure JM, et al: Premenstrual affective syndrome and affective disorder. Br J Psychiatry 127:219–221, 1975

Chapter 2

The Biology of Premenstrual Changes: What Do We Really Know?

Uriel Halbreich, M.D.
Jean Endicott, Ph.D.

Chapter 2

The Biology of Premenstrual Changes: What Do We Really Know?

T he menstrual cycle is the most apparent hormonal characteristic of women during their reproductive years. It is a mainly cyclic rhythm of the hypothalamic-pituitary-gonadal (HPG) system which is regulated by the neurotransmitters (e.g., monoamines) and neuromodulators (e.g., endorphins and prostaglandins) of the higher central nervous system (CNS). The HPG system influences the function and the structure of peripheral target organs as part of the regulation of the reproductive system.

The function of the HPG system, however, is not a one-way stream from the CNS down to the reproductive organs. There is instead an intricate and complex network of feedback mechanisms by which peripheral "stations" in the HPG axis (e.g., estrogen) participate in the regulation of the higher levels of that system (e.g., neurotransmitters and gonadotropins) and keep its dynamic rhythm in balance.

Furthermore, the female gonadal hormones, estrogens and progesterone, have been shown to influence a myriad of other systems and functions ranging from those that are putatively involved in regulation of mood and behavior, to those that influence fluid and electrolyte balance, temperature, allergies, regulation of other hormones, and many other systems.

In this chapter the possible involvement of gonadal hormones (directly or via their interaction with other biological factors) in the pathophysiology of the diverse changes occurring during the premenstrual period will be examined.

HORMONAL FLUCTUATIONS ALONG THE MENSTRUAL CYCLE

The regulation and physiology of the human menstrual cycle constitute the subject of numerous publications (Yen 1980) and will not be reviewed in detail here. The fluctuations of hormones and other biological factors along the menstrual cycle will be described mainly according to the widely accepted functional division of the menstrual cycle into a follicular, or proliferative, phase and a luteal, or secretory, phase. The follicular phase starts with the beginning of menses and ends with the ovulatory phase, which is characterized by peak levels of luteinizing hormone and follicle-stimulating hormone, follicular maturation, and ovulation. The luteal phase is characterized by progesterone secretion from the corpus luteum. Its length is more or less constant for the individual woman. In most women it lasts 14 days; however, there is some variability from one woman to another. It ends with the beginning of the following menses. The late luteal phase is also called the premenstrual period.

The pattern of secretion of hormones that were hypothesized to be associated with the premenstrual pathophysiology is presented in Figure 1. During the second half of the follicular phase there is a marked increase in plasma levels of estradiol and estrone, which reach peaks shortly before ovulation. Then there is a sharp decline which is followed by a gradual luteal increase. A few days before the beginning of menstrual bleeding, there is a sharp withdrawal of estrogen. Progesterone is almost undetectable during the follicular phase. After ovulation progesterone is secreted by the corpus luteum; the levels reach a peak shortly after the midluteal phase and then sharply decline as the menses approach. Basal body temperature follows the same pattern as progesterone. Levels of androgens, testosterone and androstenediol, are at their peak shortly before ovulation; they then decline, but just before the menses they begin to show a slight increase.

Aldosterone, which is involved in regulation of minerals and fluids, shows a small peak just prior to ovulation and a larger peak in the second half of the luteal phase when its pattern resembles that of estrogens.

There are some reports that plasma levels of prolactin (PRL) are higher during the luteal phase than during the follicular phase, but not all studies confirm this. Plasma levels of cortisol (and adrenocorticotropic hormone) were claimed to be higher during the luteal phase, but this is probably not the case. Recent studies have focused on the involvement of endorphins in the regulation of the menstrual cycle. Fluctuations in their activity and their interrelationship with the HPG axis along the menstrual cycle have been demonstrated. However, we are unaware of demonstration of cyclic fluctuations of mean plasma levels of β-endorphins or enkephalins in women. At least two groups (including ours) were unable to show such fluc-

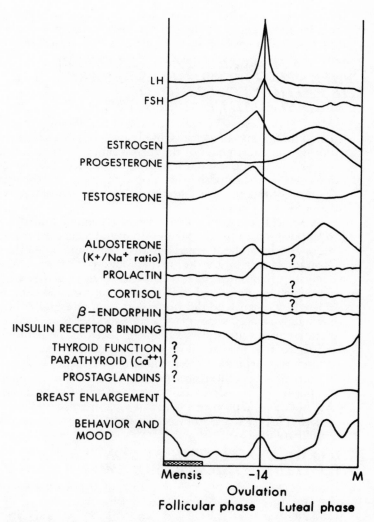

Figure 1. Hormonal Fluctuations Along the Normal Human Menstrual Cycle

tuations. The binding of insulin receptors in monocytes has been shown to be inverse to the levels of estrogens.

Surprisingly, menstrual fluctuations in some systems that may be relevant to changes in mood and behavior along the menstrual cycle have been almost ignored. For example, we are unaware of detailed studies of changes in thyroid function, calcium metabolism, and prostaglandin levels in various phases of the menstrual cycle.

THE COMMONSENSE PROCESS OF GENERATING HYPOTHESES REGARDING THE PATHOPHYSIOLOGY OF PREMENSTRUAL CHANGES (PMCs)

Many hypotheses generated to explain the etiology of PMCs were based on findings of a change in plasma levels of a specific substance during the luteal phase of the menstrual cycle. If such changes occurred during the late luteal phase (the premenstrual period) and if a change in the opposite direction took place shortly after the beginning of menses, the causative role of that substance was felt to be even more convincing.

A second step was a more detailed examination of a temporal relationship between the premenstrual and menstrual changes in levels or activity of the assumed causative factor and physical and mental changes. If such a relationship was found (which was almost always the case), then luteal or premenstrual levels of the given substance in women who reported PMCs were compared and contrasted with those in women who did not report such changes. A further, and seemingly strong, support for such hypotheses was derived from a putative involvement of a variable-in-focus in the pathophysiology of disorders similar to those occurring premenstrually (e.g., water retention or depression). A further line of evidence was derived from reports of successful treatment trials aimed at increasing levels of a "deficient" substance or blocking the activity of an excessive one. Methodological problems with this logic are discussed in detail elsewhere (Halbreich and Endicott, in press). The main hypotheses generated are discussed below.

BIOLOGICAL HYPOTHESES CONCERNING THE PATHOPHYSIOLOGY OF PMCs

Some detailed reviews of the gamut of hypotheses attempting to explain the etiology of PMC have been published recently (Rausch and Janowsky 1982; Reid and Yen 1981; Steiner and Carroll 1977). We will not duplicate their efforts and will only briefly refer to highlights of the various hypotheses. Detailed references for the data substantiating or disconfirming the hypotheses are to be found in these reviews.

Ovarian Hormones and PMCs

In seeking to explain the cause of PMC, most investigators have regarded the gonadal hormones, progesterone and estrogen, as the "natural culprits." The assumption that low luteal levels of progesterone are responsible for PMCs was and still is widely advocated. Low levels of progesterone in women with PMCs have been reported. However, there are other reports of high luteal levels of progesterone in women with PMCs. Results of treatment trials with progesterone are conflicting. Dalton treated thousands of women with progesterone, but we are unaware of any well-controlled study conducted by that pioneer in the field. Her enthusiastic propagation of the case for progesterone is more than balanced by double-blind well-controlled studies that disconfirm her claim. At best the decreased-progesterone hypothesis is still awaiting further scientific substantiation. One step further is the attribution of PMCs not to low absolute levels of progesterone but to its premenstrual decline—a possibility that may be supported by the similarity to hormonal changes during other periods in women's lives during which they may have dysphoric mood changes (e.g., postpartum "blues").

Excess of estrogen is another "suspect"; however, another frequently made suggestion is that a premenstrual decrease in estrogen levels is responsible for PMCs. The hypothesis that the main pathophysiology of PMCs is a change in estrogen-progesterone ratio, with relatively high levels of estrogen and low levels of progesterone, is probably a somewhat more sophisticated approach to understanding PMCs. However, even the ratio theory may be too simplistic. It has been demonstrated that there is a great interindividual variability of plasma levels of progesterone and estrogen among women with dysphoric PMCs. The suggestion that there are different types of PMC and that women with predominant anxiety-irritability may have high estrogen-progesterone ratios, whereas women with predominant premenstrual depression may have low estrogen-progesterone ratios, may provide a partial explanation to the high variability in hormonal levels and ratios. However, this assumption awaits better substantiation. When women are grouped according to the specific Premenstrual Assessment Form (PAF) (Halbreich et al. 1982), those with the dysphoric subtype (anxious-agitated PMCs, which presumably should be associated with high estrogen-progesterone ratio) show a wide diversity in levels of estrogen and progesterone as well as changes in the ratio. A better explanation is still needed for the multiplicity of levels of estrogen and progesterone and their ratio.

Attempts at Explanation of Fluid and Electrolyte Imbalance

Because of the prevalence of premenstrual syndromes that may be related to fluid and electrolyte imbalance, there are some hypotheses that PMCs are caused by variables that may influence such imbalance.

Increased aldosterone or renin-angiotensin activity has been suggested as an etiologic mechanism. Some authors have suggested that the increases are due to luteal increases of estrogen or progesterone or both which may cause increases in levels of plasma renin substrate (PRS), plasma renin activity (PRA), plasma angiotensin II and aldosterone. Estrogen has sodium- and water-retaining effects by itself, whereas progesterone is a natriuretic agent.

The interest in premenstrual water retention has led to a further speculation that levels of vasopressin (a hormone that promotes water retention) may be elevated premenstrually. This is an interesting suggestion because vasopressin presumably has a positive effect on memory and other cognitive functions in humans and animals. It has even been suggested that an increase in its levels may be associated with improved mood in endogenously depressed patients.

The possible association of vasopressin with PMCs raises interesting questions, especially because it implies that women with premenstrual edema due to increased vasopressin activity should have better premenstrual cognitive activity. This is contrary to usual clinical observations. We are unaware of any solid data supporting the speculation about vasopressin.

A somewhat related hypothesis is that of the involvement of PRL in PMCs. Some groups have found increased premenstrual levels of PRL in women with PMCs (mostly anxiety), but like other hypotheses concerning the etiology of PMCs, this finding has been disconfirmed by others. Results of a series of treatment studies with the dopamine agonist bromocriptine, which suppresses levels of PRL, were conflicting as well. At best, bromocriptine appears beneficial in improving water retention and related symptoms. The impact of bromocriptine on mood and behavior is still questionable, although heuristically this is an interesting issue because the alleged premenstrual increase in levels of PRL may actually be due to decreased dopaminergic activity during this period. (The possible involvement of monoamines in PMCs will be discussed later.) Bromocriptine may act through its influence on dopamine. Relatively little attention has been paid to the role of dopamine in regulation of mood and behavior, although there are some suggestions that it may play a role in regulation of activity associated with dysphoric changes. As is the case with most other biological aspects of PMCs, this is still an open question.

The Hypothalamic-Pituitary-Adrenal System (HPA)

Following the rationale that abnormal activity of the HPA system is associated with depression, it has been suggested that plasma levels of cortisol may be elevated premenstrually or that the cortisol response to stress may be higher during that period than at midcycle. Our own studies show that plasma levels of cortisol are not increased premenstrually. Further support for the lack of substantial premenstrual changes in the HPA system is derived from the finding that results of the dexamethasone-suppression test are normal in women with PMCs even when the women report severe premenstrual dysphoric changes.

Hypoglycemia

Premenstrual increased appetite, craving of sweets, dizziness, fatigue, irritability, and even some dysphoric mood changes are attributed by some to premenstrual hypoglycemia. The decrease in insulin-binding sites in monocytes during the luteal phase compared with the follicular phase, as well as the inverse relationship between receptor binding and levels of gonadal hormones, may add some support to that notion. The hypoglycemia theory of PMC is quite popular, and changes in nutrition as a treatment modality have been suggested and highly recommended, especially by trade magazines. However, we know of no well-controlled study to substantiate this theory.

Vitamins and Nutrients

Vitamin B_6 (pyridoxine) is a coenzyme in the biosynthesis of serotonin from tryptophan, its amino acid precursor. Estrogen may cause a decrease in levels of vitamin B_6 (Adams et al. 1974). Even though pyridoxine is widely used by women as treatment for PMC, its actual role is still undetermined, as are the roles of other vitamins.

The possible involvement of monoamine precursors, such as the amino acids tryptophan and tyrosine, is at present unclear. Decreased availability of these amino acids in cases of depression has been postulated. It is interesting to note that the same craving of sweets that can be used to support the hypoglycemia hypothesis can be used to support the decreased tryptophan or tyrosine hypothesis. The ratio between tryptophan and other competing amino acids may be more important than the absolute plasma levels of that amino acid. This ratio can be favorably influenced by a meal rich in carbohydrates, which causes a decrease in plasma levels of leucine, valine, and isoleucine (the "competing amino acids"), thus increasing the availability of tryptophan to the brain. Hence, the craving of food rich in carbohydrates may be viewed as a subconscious attempt at self-help by advocates of several different hypotheses.

The influence of quantities of plasma estrogen and progesterone on levels of these amino acids is unknown. No one has studied the question of whether there are or are not fluctuations of their levels during the menstrual cycle. Differences in the levels or ratios between women with PMCs and those without them also remain to be studied.

Deficiency or Withdrawal of Endorphins

The involvement of endorphins in the pathophysiology of PMCs has been suggested. The rationale for this hypothesis (like those for many other hypotheses on PMCs) is derived from the postulated inter-relationship between ovarian hormones and endorphins (based mostly on animal studies of basal levels and on administration of naloxone, an endorphin antagonist, in humans). The rationale is also based on the postulated influence of endorphins on mood and behavior and on the symptoms accompanying their withdrawal. The influence of endorphins on other systems further enhances the interest in their possible involvement in PMCs. In two studies, including our own, no fluctuation related to the menstrual cycle was found in mean group levels of β-endorphin. However, when individual cases are examined, there may be a temporal association between decreased levels of β-endorphin and low energy. The question of whether this observation is of significance awaits further collection of data.

Other Hypotheses Concerning the Etiology of PMCs

A score of hypotheses concerning the etiology of PMCs have been suggested: allergies to various substances and excesses or deficiencies of peptides, such as melanocyte-stimulating hormone, trace amines, such as phenylethylamine, melatonin, prostaglandins, and many others. At this point some of the suggested models are interesting and theoretically convincing. However, they have not been tested, and in most cases the data brought to support them are tangential and indirect. The models provide an open field for interested researchers.

MONOAMINES AND THE PATHOPHYSIOLOGY OF PMCs

As is demonstrated in Figure 2, various indicators of activity of monoamines have been shown to change premenstrually. It may be suggested that the changes in activity of noradrenergic, serotonergic, and cholinergic systems are comparable to similar changes found in subgroups of patients with depressive disorders. These changes in activity of monoamines may be related to premenstrual changes in ovarian hormones, more specifically to decreased levels of estrogen and progesterone. The interaction between steroid hormones and neurotransmitters has been reviewed elsewhere (McEwen et al., in

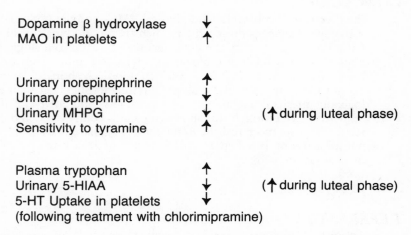

Figure 2. Premenstrual Changes in Variables Related to Monoamine Transmitters (MAO indicates monoamine oxidase; MHPG indicates 3-methoxy-4-hydroxyphenylglycol; 5-HIAA indicates 5-hydroxy-indoleacetic acid; 5-HT indicates 5-hydroxytryptamine)

press). A possible involvement of monoamines in premenstrual water and fluid imbalance was reviewed by Reid and Yen (1981), and their possible involvement in premenstrual dysphoric changes was reviewed by Rausch and Janowsky (1982). We will only note here that estrogen has been shown to influence enzymes, biosynthesis, uptake, turnover, and receptors of monoamine systems in a way that is compatible with an increase in their activity or, in the case of postsynaptic receptors, in a way that is compatible with a hypothesized antidepressant effect. The same can be shown for progesterone, which may have a depressant effect. Hence, the premenstrual decrease in levels of ovarian hormones may be associated with changes in monoamines that, in turn, are involved with the pathophysiology of PMCs.

At present the hypothesis that changes in monoamines—in conjunction with changes in ovarian hormones—are involved in the etiology of PMCs is very attractive and testable. Further elucidation of that hypothesis, with an emphasis on the multivariate PMCs, is to be found in a previous publication (Halbreich and Endicott 1982). Methodological issues are also elaborated elsewhere (Halbreich and Endicott, in press).

CONCLUSION

The diversity of behavioral and physical PMCs and the multiplicity of biological changes during the premenstrual period make it likely that attempting to relate the entire gamut of PMCs to a single biological factor will fail. A multivariate approach is more likely to be fruitful for the study of PMCs. Such an approach should take into account the changes of the multiple interrelationships between endogenous mechanisms, individual vulnerability, and environmental influences. Even though this approach sounds complicated and difficult, it may be more realistic in the same way that a statue with its multidimensions is a better representation of reality than a two-dimensional drawing.

REFERENCES

Halbreich U, Endicott J: Future directions in the study of premenstrual changes. Psychopharmacol Bull 18:121–123, 1982

Halbreich U, Endicott J, Schacht S, et al: The diversity of premenstrual changes as reflected in the Premenstrual Assessment Form. Acta Psychiatr Scand 64:46–65, 1982

Halbreich U, Endicott J: Methodological issues in studies of premenstrual changes. Psychoneuroendocrinology (in press)

McEwen BS, Biegon A, Fischette CT, et al: Toward a neurochemical basis of steroid hormones action, in Frontiers in Neuroendocrinology. Edited by Ganong WF, Mortons L. New York, Raven Press, 1984

Rausch JL, Janowsky DS: Premenstrual tension: etiology, in Behavior and the Menstrual Cycle. Edited by Freidman R. New York, Marcel Dekker, 1982

Reid R, Yen SSC: Premenstrual syndrome. Am J Obstet Gynecol 139:85–104, 1981

Steiner M, Carroll BJ: The psychobiology of premenstrual dysphoria: review of theories and treatments. Psychoneuroendocrinology 2:321–335, 1977

Yen SS: Neuroendocrine regulation of the menstrual cycle, in Neuroendocrinology. Edited by Krieger DT, Hughes JC. Sanderland, Mass, Sinauer Association, 1980, pp 259–272

Chapter 3

Menstrually Related Mood Disorders

David R. Rubinow, M.D.
Peter Roy-Byrne, M.D.
M. Christine Hoban, M.S.W.
Gay N. Grover, M.S.N.
Robert M. Post, M.D.

Chapter 3

Menstrually Related Mood Disorders

T
he area of menstrually related mood disorders is characterized by conceptual promise and clinical controversy. Although the relationship between mood and menstruation has interested phenomenologists for centuries, no conclusive evidence exists with respect to the etiology or treatment of the menstrually related mood syndromes largely because of the methodologic confusion displayed by investigators in this field. This chapter will briefly summarize some of the historical data suggesting a relationship between disorders of mood and behavior and menstrual cycle phase, propose an operational definition for a menstrually related disorder, review the extent to which questions inherent in that definition have been addressed in the literature, describe the prospective use of an analogue scale rating instrument, and discuss possible relationships between premenstrual syndromes and formal psychiatric disorders. The intent of this chapter is to suggest that the practical and theoretical importance of this area requires careful research efforts instead of anecdotal reports and ideological conviction.

HISTORICAL REVIEW

Reference to major changes in mood and behavior in relation to menstrual cycle phase appears as early as the *Sickness of Virgins* by Hippocrates (Simon 1978). Levitical law viewed menstruation as a "crisis period" during which intercourse should be prohibited (Sutherland 1892). The Talmud warned that a child conceived during menstruation would become mentally unstable and/or morally degenerate (Sutherland 1892). In more modern times, Pinel (1799) reported a case of menstrually related depression, and Esquirol, Morel, Greissinger, and Sutherland (Sutherland 1892) all described manic excitement confined to the catamenial period with occasional instances of mania associated with the premenstruum or suppression of menses. Icard, in *La Femme Pendant La Periode Menstruelle* (1890), attributed an impressive list of mood and behavioral disturbances, including homicidal or suicidal mania, delirious insanity, hallucinations, and melancholia, to disorders of menstruation. According to Icard,

> . . . the menstrual function can by sympathy, especially in those predisposed, create a mental condition varying from a simple psychalgia, that is to say, a simple moral malaise, a simple troubling of the soul, to actual insanity, to a complete loss of reason, and modifying the acts of a women from simple weakness to absolute irresponsibility. (page 266)

With the description by Robert Frank of "premenstrual tension" (1931), interest in the relationship between mood/behavior and menstruation became exclusively focused on the premenstrual tension syndrome or the premenstrual syndrome(s). Despite the wealth of clinical descriptions the absence of a clearly stated, testable definition of menstrually related syndromes has greatly compromised efforts to explore and understand the nature of this biobehavioral disorder.

METHODOLOGICAL ISSUES

For clinical research as well as clinical practice, the first question that must be posed is, How do you define that which you wish to study (or treat)? One can operationally define a menstrually related mood disorder as the cyclic recurrence of symptoms that are of sufficient severity so as to interfere with certain aspects of life and that occur with a consistent and predictable relationship to menstruation. Several derivative questions are inherent in this definition.

(1) What are the symptoms that are experienced? The list of symptoms that have been attributed to the premenstrual syndrome is astounding. Practically any symptom that one might expect to encounter in a general medical practice has in one study or another been described as a feature of premenstrual syndrome. Halbreich et al. (1982) have attempted to deal with this diversity of symptoms by designing the Premenstrual Assessment Form, with which they hope to identify clinically meaningful symptom clusters or subsyndromes that can be defined with the use of mutually exclusive symptom components. As these authors appropriately caution, their subsyndromes must at present be viewed as descriptors rather than diagnoses.

(2) To what degree are the symptoms experienced, i.e., what is their intensity? Problems related to this question have included the failure of investigators to measure symptom severity (Sutherland and Stew-

art 1965), attribution of clinical significance to statistically significant but clinically insubstantial changes (Taylor 1979), and utilization of an insensitive severity measure or one that is categorical rather than dimensional and therefore more subject to perceptual bias (Abraham 1980).

(3) When do symptoms occur in relationship to menstruation?

(4) What is the symptomatic baseline upon which symptoms fluctuate?

These two questions are absolutely critical to the definition of premenstrual syndromes, for it is the linkage of symptoms to menstrual cycle phase that defines them as "menstrually related" or "premenstrual." Yet it is precisely the timing of symptom occurrence that has paradoxically received the least attention. Thus, not only is there great variability in the usage of the term "premenstrual" but there is also surprisingly little attempt made to describe the symptomatic baseline against which premenstrual symptoms must be measured. Premenstrual symptoms must be evaluated in the context of the remainder of the menstrual cycle in order to be able to distinguish successfully among premenstrual appearance of symptoms, premenstrual exacerbation of preexisting symptoms, and premenstrual continuation of symptoms.

The major problem underlying most studies of premenstrual syndromes, aside from the multitude of populations examined, is the use of inadequate methods to select subjects and evaluate symptoms. Despite numerous demonstrations that retrospective ratings are not generally validated by daily prospective ratings and, in fact, overestimate symptoms experienced (McCance et al. 1937; Abplanalp et al. 1979; Sampson and Prescott 1981), most studies to date have used retrospective reports of menstrually related symptoms as the sole entry criterion without prospectively confirming the existence of the relationship between symptom occurrence and menstruation.

PROSPECTIVE ASSESSMENT

As part of our attempt to study menstrually related mood disorders, we sought a mood rating method that would permit prospective confirmation of the relationship between mood and menstruation. We selected as our rating instrument a 100-mm line visual analogue scale, as this rating method appears to confer many advantages over conventional scales in rating subjective feeling (Bond and Lader 1974; Aitken 1969). Following completion of two months of daily ratings, the visual analogue scales were graphed (Figures 1 and 2), and a menstrually related mood syndrome was defined as at least a 30 percent increase in mean negative mood rating score during the week prior to menstruation compared with the week following the

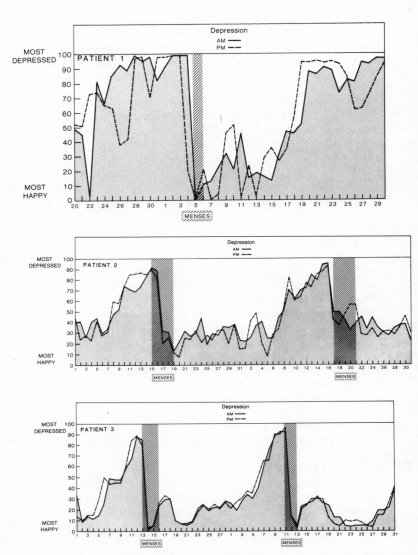

Figure 1. Depression Self-Ratings of Three Women with Menstrually Related Mood Disorders

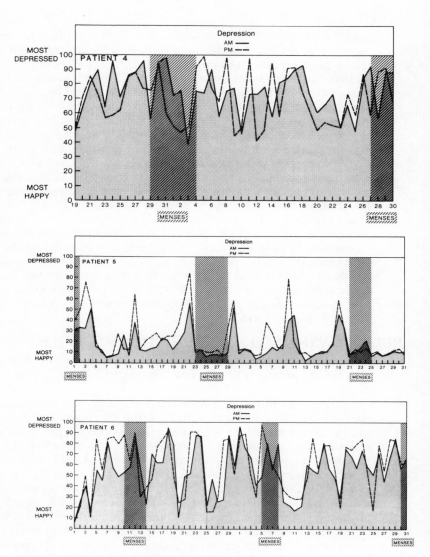

Figure 2. Depression Self-Ratings of Three Women Without Menstrually Related Mood Disorders

cessation of menstruation. A similar definition was proposed and endorsed by the National Institute of Mental Health premenstrual syndrome research workshop.

Of the first 160 women who self-referred for participation in our premenstrual syndrome program and who completed three months of prospective ratings, 69 (43 percent) provided clear evidence of a menstrually related mood disorder. This finding not only demonstrates the utility of a prospective rating method for identifying subjects for participation in clinical studies but also suggests that those studies that select subjects solely on the basis of a history of premenstrual syndrome without prospective confirmation include a substantial number of subjects who either do not have premenstrual syndrome or have a concurrent disorder that accounts for far more of the variability in their mood than does any menstrually related disorder. Subjects with prospectively confirmed premenstrual syndrome were by history clinically indistinguishable from those lacking prospective evidence of premenstrual syndrome. It appears then that prospective longitudinal rating methods may provide greater diagnostic homogeneity and permit determination of the practical and conceptual significance of the relationship between menstruation and disorders of mood and behavior.

RELATIONSHIP TO PSYCHIATRIC DISORDERS

There are at least four major questions that address the relationship between menstrually related mood changes and formal psychiatric disorder.

(1) Are major psychiatric syndromes and premenstrual syndromes concurrent but separate disorders? A number of attempts have been made to describe the prevalence of premenstrual disorders in patients with major psychiatric disorders. Four groups have reported a two-thirds prevalence of premenstrual affective syndrome in patients with a history of major affective disorder (Endicott et al. 1981; Kashiwagi et al. 1976; Diamond et al. 1976; Hurt et al. 1982). Attempts have also been made to describe the prevalence of psychiatric disorders in women with premenstrual syndromes. Among the subjects from five different samples meeting Endicott and Halbreich's criteria for premenstrual "full depressive syndrome," 57 percent to 100 percent had a lifetime diagnosis of major depressive disorder in contrast to only zero to 20 percent with no history of mental illness (Halbreich and Endicott, submitted for publication). In all of the above-mentioned studies, the diagnosis of premenstrual syndrome was made on the basis of retrospective data, with the exception of a small number of patients ($n = 10$) in Halbreich and Endicott's study. For

this group with prospectively confirmed premenstrual syndrome, the reported prevalence of history of a major depressive disorder was 60 percent.

Our examination of life history of psychiatric illness, as determined from the Schedule for Affective Disorder and Schizophrenia–Lifetime interview, showed significant differences in women with premenstrual syndrome (PMS+) and those without prospectively confirmed menstrually related mood disorder (PMS−) ($\chi^2 = 10.57$, $p < .005$) (DeJong et al., submitted for publication). The major difference between these two groups is the very high proportion of PMS− patients with a past history of psychiatric disorder (21/24, 88 percent) compared with PMS+ patients (15/33, 45 percent). Thus, while the percentage of the PMS+ group with a history of psychiatric disorder is somewhat greater than that found in the general population, the lifetime psychiatric history of those complaining of premenstrual syndrome but lacking prospective evidence of same (PMS−) is extremely high (DeJong et al., submitted for publication). This illustrates the danger of inferring the prevalence of psychiatric morbidity in women with premenstrual syndrome from studies using solely retrospective diagnostic techniques and therefore utilizing heterogenous samples that are not representative of the population with premenstrual syndrome. The difference between the 60 percent prevalence rate of history of major depressive disorder reported by Halbreich and Endicott and the 45 percent rate for lifetime history of psychiatric disorder that we observed may reflect differences in sampling selection or in sample size ($n = 10$ vs. $n = 33$, respectively).

(2) Can premenstrual symptoms mimic major psychiatric disorders, or do these symptoms represent premenstrual intensification or recurrence of major psychiatric syndromes? This question addresses the need to distinguish among symptom occurrence, exacerbation, recrudescence, and clustering. Although there are many reports of "premenstrual tension associated with psychotic episodes" (Williams and Weekes 1952) or "mental illness aligned with the menstrual cycle" (Endo et al. 1978), the terms describing the relationship between psychiatric symptoms and menstruation are frequently imprecisely used. It is the baseline symptoms or absence of symptoms that determine whether psychiatric symptoms are "associated with" or exacerbated during the premenstruum. Similarly, a previously experienced psychiatric syndrome that reappears solely in the luteal phase may represent a menstrually linked recrudescence of the psychiatric syndrome, whereas the premenstrual worsening of continuously experienced pscyhiatric symptoms represents menstrually linked exacerbation of psychiatric syndromes. The experience of episodic disorders (e.g., panic or bu-

limic episodes) solely in the context of the luteal phase, premenstrual symptom clustering, has been reported but not objectively confirmed.

(3) Is premenstrual syndrome a sensitizing experience that may influence the course or development of a major psychiatric syndrome? Menstrually related mood changes might influence the evolution of psychiatric disorders by serving as sensitizing stimuli. Studies of cocaine sensitization and amygdala kindling have demonstrated that repetitive administration of a subictal chemical or electrical stimulus can produce increasing effects and profound long-term changes in brain activity and behavior (Post and Ballenger 1981). The repetitive experience of premenstrual dysphoria might therefore, in individuals who are genetically predisposed, allow for the gradual development or expression of an affective illness based on these sensitization-like mechanisms. The report by Price (1980) of temporal lobe epilepsy presenting as a premenstrual affective syndrome is consistent with both the state model of symptom expression as well as the sensitization model of symptom development. Longitudinal study of the course of menstrually related disorders may help to clarify further the relevance of the sensitization model to these disorders as well as their relationship to major psychiatric disorders.

(4) Is there etiologic commonality between menstrual mood syndromes and major psychiatric syndromes that might allow one to serve as a model for exploration of the other? The occurrence of major endocrine changes, limbic dysregulation, and fluid and electrolyte disturbances in association with both psychiatric and menstrually related mood disorders suggest that further study of the intimate relationship between menstrual cycle physiology and central nervous system activity may help expand our understanding of the neurobiology of both types of disorders as well as the relationship between them. One model that may help organize clinical observations of the menstrually related mood disorders is the state model of psychological functioning (Horowitz 1979) which suggests that the normal human condition comprises a variety of well-differentiated experiential or behavioral states that are characterized by specific attitudes, ideas, memories, affects, perceptions, and self and object relations. These states are recurrent and internally consistent and therefore describable and predictable. According to this model, premenstrual syndrome is not a symptom-specific disturbance but is rather a disorder characterized by a menstrual cycle–linked transition into a particular experiential state, usually, but not exclusively, dysphoric in nature. By carefully studying the "switch," or the point of premenstrual-state transition, we may better understand the process by which biology influences the tran-

sition between experiential states and thereby enhance our knowledge of normal as well as pathological human functioning.

CONCLUSIONS

The influence of menstrual cycle phase upon mood change is not only of practical relevance (as a factor that may influence the course of treatment of patients) but is, in addition, heuristically useful (as a model for learning about changes in mental-emotional state) and conceptually important (as a potential means for exploring the relationship between biological rhythms and psychiatric phenomenology). Advances in neurobiology as well as the utilization of more precise, prospective, longitudinal evaluative methods may allow research into premenstrual syndrome to greatly advance our understanding of the regulation of mood in normal states and pathological conditions.

REFERENCES

Abplanalp JM, Donnelly AF, Rose RM: Psychoendocrinology of menstrual cycle. I. enjoyment of daily activities and moods. Psychosom Med 41:587–604, 1979

Abraham GE: The premenstrual tension syndromes, in Contemporary Obstetric and Gynecologic Nursing, vol 3. Edited by McNall LK. St. Louis, C.V. Mosby, 1980

Aitken RCB: Measurement of feelings using visual analogue scales. Proc R Soc Med 62:989–992, 1969

Bond A, Lader M: The use of analogue scales in rating subjective feelings. Br J Med Psychol 47:211–218, 1974

Diamond SB, Rubinstein AA, Dunner DL, et al: Menstrual problems in women with primary affective illness. Compr Psychiatry 17:541–548, 1976

Endicott J, Halbreich U, Schacht S, et al: Premenstrual changes and affective disorders. Psychosom Med 43:519–529, 1981

Endo M, Daiguji M, Asano Y, et al: Periodic psychosis recurring in association with menstrual cycle. J Clin Psychiatry 39:456–466, 1978

Frank RT: The hormonal causes of premenstrual tension. Archives of Neurology and Psychiatry 26:1053–1057, 1931

Halbreich U, Endicott J, Schacht S, et al: The diversity of premenstrual changes as reflected in the premenstrual assessment form. Acta Psychiatr Scand 65:46–65, 1982

Halbreich U, Endicott J, Nee J: Premenstrual depressive changes: value of differentiation. Arch Gen Psychiatry 40:525–542, 1983

Horowitz M: States of Mind. New York, Plenum Press, 1979

Hurt SW, Freidman RC, Clarkin J, et al: Psychopathology in the menstrual cycle, in Behavior and the Menstrual Cycle. Edited by Freidman RC, New York, Marcel Dekker, 1982

Icard S: La Femme Pandant La Periode Menstruelle. Paris, Felix Alcan, 1890

Kashiwagi T, McClure JM Jr, Wetzel RD: Premenstrual affective syndrome and psychiatric disorder. Dis Nerv Syst 37:116–119, 1976

McCance RA, Luff RC, Widdowson E: Physical and emotional periodicity in women. J Hyg (Lond) 37:571–611, 1937

Pinel P: Nosographie philosophique ou la methode de l'analyse appliqué à la medicine. Paris, Maradan, 1799

Post R, Ballenger JC: Kindling models for the progression development of behavioral psychopathology: Sensitization to electrical, pharmacological and psychological stimuli, in Handbook of Biological Psychiatry, part IV. Edited by Van Praag HM, Lader MH, Rafaelsen OJ, et al. New York, Marcel Dekker, 1981

Price, TRP: Temporal lobe epilepsy as a premenstrual behavioral syndrome. Biol Psychol 15:957–963, 1980

Rubinow DR, Roy-Byrne P, Hoban MC: Prospective assessment of menstrually related mood disorders. Am J Psychiatry 141:684–686, 1984

Sampson JA, Prescott P: The assessment of the symptoms of premenstrual syndrome and their response to therapy. Br J Psychiatry 138:399–405, 1981

Simon B: Mind and Madness in Ancient Greece. Ithaca, New York, Cornell University Press, 1978, p 243

Sutherland H: Menstruation and insanity, in A Dictionary of Psychological Medicine. Edited by Tuke, DH. Philadelphia, P. Blakistone, Son & Co, 1892

Sutherland H, Stewart I: A critical analysis of premenstrual syndrome. Lancet 1:1180–1183, 1965

Taylor JW: The timing of menstruation-related symptoms assessed by a daily symptom rating scale. Acta Psychiatr Scand 60:87–105, 1979

Williams EY, Weekes LR: Premenstrual tension associated with psychotic episodes. J Nerv Ment Dis 116:321–329, 1952

Chapter 4

Psychiatric and Gynecological Evaluation and Management of Premenstrual Symptoms

Howard J. Osofsky, M.D., Ph.D.
William Keppel, M.D.

Chapter 4

Psychiatric and Gynecological Evaluation and Management of Premenstrual Symptoms

Since the initial description of premenstrual tension by Frank in 1931, a number of etiological explanations, evaluation protocols, and strategies for treatment have been offered in an attempt to understand and alleviate premenstrual symptoms. Contributing to the discouragement of clinicians and researchers, most of the hypotheses and treatment regimens have not stood the test of time. In general, studies have been poorly designed; patient selection has been confounded by nonverified retrospective data and questionable inclusion criteria; double-blind crossover studies have not been carried out; placebo effects have not been sufficiently considered; mechanisms of hormonal interaction and treatment success or failure have been proposed, but not sufficiently tested; follow-up has been inadequate; and results have not been replicated. In addition, measurements utilized have sometimes been inappropriate. Psychological measures have not always been valid for the symptoms being studied, and endocrine assays, when performed, have often been indirect and reflective of peripheral rather than target levels of the substances assessed. Frequently, evaluation and treatment strategies have been based upon questionable theoretical frameworks. In recent years, serious attempts have been undertaken to provide scientifically sound evaluation and management efforts. At present, these efforts remain in the early stages, and they are not sufficient to provide clear clinical directions.

Other chapters in this book address theoretical underpinnings, research strategies, and treatment approaches for severe psychiatric symptoms that appear entrained with or exacerbated by the menstrual cycle. In the present chapter, we will consider clinical approaches to the evaluation and treatment of mild and moderate symptoms that may be encountered by psychiatrists and obstetricians-gynecologists. We emphasize at this point, as we will throughout the chapter, that the treatment regimens that we will describe, although frequently employed, have not in general been verified by double-blind crossover studies. However, since a number of them are in wide use at this time, it would seem worthwhile to try to understand the rationale for such approaches and some of the clinical considerations in their use. We recognize that further theoretically and methodologically sound studies are needed and that when they are carried out they will probably influence and change evaluation and treatment strategies.

DEFINITIONS AND PATTERNS OF SYMPTOMS

The first step in evaluation is clarity as to what is being evaluated. Our definition of premenstrual syndromes agrees with those stated in other chapters in this monograph. Premenstrual syndromes must have a cyclic component that is related to the menstrual cycle. The symptoms must be recurrent, usually in two out of three cycles. There also must be an interval—usually within the follicular phase of the cycle—in which the woman is either free of symptoms or shows marked improvement.

Estimates indicate that most women have some premenstrual symptoms; in various reports the range is between 20 and 90 percent; between 3 and 15 percent have severe symptoms. Rubinow (1984) has listed a number of the common symptoms of premenstrual syndromes. He has described affective, cognitive, pain, neurovegetative, autonomic, central nervous system, fluid-electrolyte, dermatological, and behavioral symptoms. Perhaps in a somewhat more simplified framework, one can divide the symptoms into those of a physical and those of an emotional nature. Obviously, there is considerable overlap. Under such a schema, physical symptoms would include the following: those of an allergic nature; gastrointestinal symptoms including food cravings, constipation, and diarrhea; lower abdominal and pelvic discomfort and bloating; joint and muscle discomfort and stiffness; pain and swelling in the breasts; and a variety of nervous system complaints such as headache, clumsiness, difficulties with concentration and memory, and seizures. Emotional symptoms would include the following: mood swings; irritability; anxiety; depression, sometimes with suicidal ideations; difficulties with control, at times including violence; eating patterns suggestive of bulimia; and psychoses. Patients may report increases or decreases in levels of energy and sexual desire; outbursts and fluctuations of symptoms may provide further confusion and distress for the patients.

In addition, premenstrual syndromes are usually described as being age related, with increasing symptoms in the late twenties, thirties, and forties. In our experience, in patients with severe emotional symptoms, there appears to be less of an age relationship to the development of symptoms. Early symptoms in adolescence may be related to earlier onset of menarche; as with older patients there is not a clear relationship to regularity of the menstrual cycle. In young women the symptoms appear less related to the symptoms of the patient's mothers but more related to lack of preparation and to the mother's expectations of symptoms. As pointed out by others in this book, there appear to be links between emotional symptoms that are related to the menstrual cycle and emotional symptoms that are related to other important events in the female reproductive life cycle, for example, postpartum depression and menopausal depression. In our experience, a number of patients report a worsening of symptoms during the first several months to one year following tubal ligation. In general, premenstrual symptoms and dysmenorrhea should be seen as separate symptoms that are somewhat unrelated. In high-quality gynecologically oriented evaluation programs, significant percentages of patients with severe symptoms appear to have emotional components to their symptoms. The corollary is also true: Patients with predominantly emotional symptoms may have physical or physiologically determined components to their symptoms.

ETIOLOGY

A number of theories have been put forth to explain the etiology of premenstrual syndromes. Chapters 2 and 3 in this volume deal with this area in depth. Therefore, although it is an important topic, we will not attempt to deal with it in the present chapter.

EVALUATION

Prospective Ratings

As has been done by others, we would like to stress that the first, and perhaps most important, step in the management with patients with premenstrual symptoms is a careful evaluation. Because of our setting, many of the patients referred to us have severe psychiatric symptoms and are in need of hospitalization and early treatment. However, we believe that it is important, when possible, to obtain a careful initial history and then prospectively follow the patient's symptoms for three months prior to instituting treatment per se. We have designed four forms that we use to have patients rate severity of symptoms prospectively in relation to daily stresses, ovulation, and menstruation. We also utilize the visual analogue scales developed by Rubinow, as well as the symptom, personal, and family and medical history forms that are being used in a number of other centers.

It would seem important to emphasize the value of the three months of prospective ratings. In our experience, as well as that of others, approximately 50 percent of the patients either drop out or require no further treatment by the end of this time interval. After preliminary discussions and initial general advice, some women describe learning self-treatment techniques as they chart their symptoms and the factors that appear to trigger the worsening of symptoms. For example, women may come to sense that whereas they crave sweets, caffeine, cigarettes, and/or alcohol, their symptoms worsen following this self-medication. Some learn that exercise on a regular basis appears to decrease these symptoms. Women become aware of triggering factors and events in their lives, and they learn some obvious remedies. For example, one woman described how visits from her overly critical mother-in-law would worsen symptoms, and she learned to invite her mother-in-law to visit at other times of the menstrual cycle. A number of women described how stressors at work were more difficult at this time, and they learned to program their work events and schedule in a way that allowed them to complete tasks and to schedule events in a more comfortable manner. Some recognized that particular marital patterns or interactions with children could create problems, and they developed techniques for avoiding or dealing with these difficulties. Another group describing their ongoing symptoms simply felt that things were under better control owing to newfound predictabilities, and they no longer felt the need for further workup. It has been our sense that for a number of the women, having professionals who were available and caring and who were acknowledging the legitimacy of their symptoms served to diminish the urgency of the symptoms and allowed for improved self-care techniques of coping with them. Thus, a category of patients exists who can learn to accept and live with their symptoms productively, the prospective symptom study period itself has a therapeutic effect.

At the end of the three-month interval, we have noted a number of different patterns. For example, some women appear to have significant symptoms, but the symptoms are apparently unrelated to the menstrual cycle (Figure 1). We estimate that this may be the pattern in approximately 50 percent of the women (which generally agrees with the results of other studies) and that such women may benefit from further psychiatric or medical evaluation and treatment. Among the remaining women a number of different pictures have emerged, and we are currently questioning the meaning of these

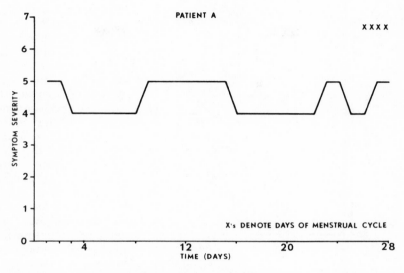

Figure 1. Depressed Feelings Varying Independently of the Menstrual Cycle in One Patient

symptoms (Figures 2–4). For example, what are different implications when women go from no symptoms to mild symptoms, as opposed to going from no symptoms to severe symptoms? What are the differential meanings—to give but a few examples—of symptoms that gradually escalate for several days prior to the period and then cease abruptly on the day when flow begins, as opposed to symptoms that continue through the period, as opposed to symptoms that are present only during the period, as opposed to symptoms that begin at ovulation then decrease and then resume prior to menstruation, as opposed to symptoms that begin at ovulation and continue unabated until menstruation? What are the differential meanings of symptoms that occur with no apparent baseline psychiatric difficulty as opposed to those that suggest an addition to, exacerbation of, or a worsening of an underlying difficulty. On the basis of current endocrinological and neuroendocrinological knowledge, it is hard to reconcile these different patterns as belonging to a single syndrome.

Evaluation of Symptoms Related to the Menstrual Cycle

For those women who have significant symptoms related to the menstrual cycle, our workup consists of the following evaluations

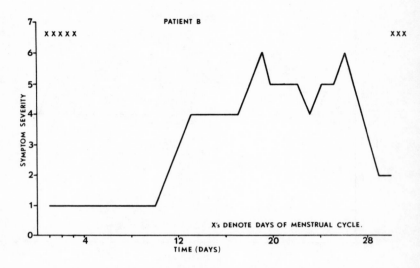

Figure 2. Depressed Feelings Varying in Relation to the Menstrual Cycle in One Patient

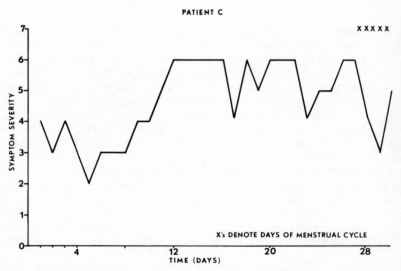

Figure 3. Depressed Feelings Possibly Varying in Relation to the Menstrual Cycle in One Patient

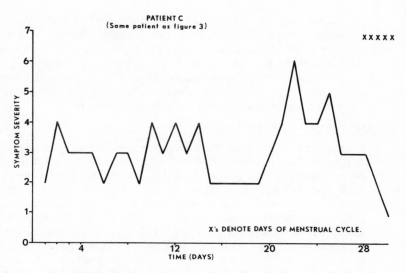

Figure 4. Suicidal Feelings Varying in Relation to the Menstrual Cycle of One Patient

that are scheduled at the height of symptoms, with repeat evaluations taking place as indicated during a symptom-free interval:

(1) Psychiatric assessments. Perhaps it almost goes without saying that we take a careful history of the symptoms, their duration, and precipitating factors; associated psychiatric symptoms including typical and atypical vegetative components; alcohol and drug use patterns; prior treatment approaches and outcome; and a review of family relationships, menstrual difficulties and psychiatric—especially affective—disorders.

(2) Medical evaluation. This includes a full medical history and physical examination, including a pelvic examination. Special emphasis is placed upon possible endocrinological, metabolic, neurological, and gynecological disorders.

(3) Psychological testing. We utilize a standard battery, as well as a Thematic Apperception Test, Rorschach test, Wechsler Adult Intelligence Scale, and other assessments as indicated.

(4) Nutritional assessment. This includes typical daily dietary patterns, with additional emphasis on areas of deficiency and other abnormalities that might be related to premenstrual symptoms.

(5) *Laboratory tests.* These include a complete blood count, blood chemistry profile, urinalysis, blood sugar analysis, T_3 and T_4 levels, TRH-stimulation test, dexamethasone suppression test, vitamin B_6 and magnesium levels, estradiol, progesterone, and prolactin levels, Papanicolaou smear with assessment for hormonal status, and, depending on neurological and cognitive symptoms, EEG and neurometric assessments.

SOME OVERALL FINDINGS

Consistent with the data of Brooks-Gunn and Ruble (personal communication) and Ruble (1984) we have noted a greater relationship between the patient's symptoms and her mother's attitudes and other background characteristics than between the patient's symptoms and her mother's symptoms. A number of patients, especially those with significant symptoms that appear sporadically or throughout the menstrual cycle, have demonstrated underlying psychiatric difficulty. In a number of patients with severe symptoms, mixed or borderline personality disorders have been diagnosed. Consistent with the descriptions of Rubinow and Roy-Byrne (1984) and Endicott et al. (1981), affective components have been prominent; in some cases, they have appeared entrained with, or exacerbated by, the menstrual cycle. A variety of gynecological difficulties may be linked with physical symptoms, and menstrual irregularity may accompany, or be influenced by, emotional symptoms. Links between gynecological difficulty and the etiology of emotional symptoms have been less clearly apparent. On psychological testing an increase in dependency needs has been especially prominent, and this may be related to the improvement in symptoms when the patients enter into a therapeutic relationship. We have now seen four patients in whom EEG or neurometric patterns have evidenced differences related to the menstrual cycle. Of some note, the differences corresponded to the patients' symptoms. This is consistent with the reports of catamenial epilepsy noted in the literature (Newmark and Penrey 1980). To date, we have been disappointed in the findings from the dexamethasone suppression test, the TRH-stimulation test, and, in general, the estradiol and progesterone determinations. We are currently considering performing the dexamethasone suppression test and TRH-stimulation test only when clinically indicated and are considering the possibility of using different hormonal assessments.

TREATMENT

In this section we will focus on hormonal and other medical approaches to treatment. Other authors in this book, for example Glick, discuss the role of psychotropic medications in detail. We would also emphasize that when evaluation reveals an underlying psychiatric difficulty, even with some worsening of symptoms premenstrually, the underlying emotional difficulty should be treated with the most appropriate psychiatric regimen, whether it be psychotherapy, family therapy, psychopharmacological agents, or a combination of these interventions. We approach this section with some trepidation because of the paucity of good double-blind, placebo-controlled, cross-over studies. Medications are currently being prescribed with questionable theoretical rationale and without confirmatory data related to absorption patterns, outcome, or follow-up. Furthermore, medications are being prescribed without approval by the Food and Drug Administration. Yet we are respectful of the fact that good clinicians have the sense that some medications are of benefit in at least some cases. Furthermore, and as is described by Glick, there has been a sense that in individuals or small groups of cases adding such medications to a psychotropic regimen has, on occasion, been useful.

It would seem important to emphasize that at this time with the fragmentary knowledge at hand, there is no one answer or no right answer. Therefore it would be advisable for clinicians to be cautious if they are prescribing medications, to use the approaches that appear to be pharmacologically safest, and to leave more experimental approaches for last. In most good programs, clinicians do not promise patients a cure but tell patients that they will try to help with their symptoms. Clinicians should be encouraged to follow patients carefully, to look for side effects, to be open to the possibility of failures, and to assess the need for alternative approaches. Because there is currently no standard treatment, patients at times may seek treatment from advocates of a specific regimen. Unfortunately, some patients have reported that they have been afraid or found it difficult to discuss poor treatment results of enthusiastically promoted programs. It is important to know about complications, failures, and the return or worsening of symptoms; lack of knowledge about such outcomes is likely to have inappropriate influences on clinicians' future approaches to treatment.

With this in mind, we will summarize some current approaches that are commonly used for treatment. We again emphasize that methodologically sound data are not present to substantiate clearly the efficacy of various treatment regimens and that with further research studies, better theoretical and clinical understandings may be possible in the coming years (Rubinow and Roy-Byrne 1984). Yet, we recognize that many women are currently requesting treatment for symptoms related to the menstrual cycle and that clinicians are prescribing treatment. For that reason, we will offer some guidelines for those occasions when treatment seems necessary to the clinician.

Initial General Approaches

As we have indicated, whenever possible we begin with a regimen that incorporates exercise, a well-balanced diet—including decreased intake of refined sugars, coffee, tea, and chocolate—and decreased alcohol consumption prior to and during the time of the symptoms. We encourage women to decrease or discontinue smoking. There is a logical rationale to encouraging regular exercise in that exercise appears to affect endorphin balance (Carr et al. 1981), and endorphins have recently been postulated as playing an etiologic role in premenstrual syndrome (Reid and Yen 1983). Although hypoglycemic patterns have not been demonstrated in association with premenstrual syndrome, we believe that based on studies of endocrinologically related variations in glucose utilization, the dietary recommendations also have some rationale (Bertoli et al. 1980). If possible, we attempt to help women to identify and control stressors that appear to trigger symptoms. We recognize the biasing factors in the types of women who are referred to us; however, in our experience a considerable number of women appear to benefit from individual psychotherapy, family therapy, or both.

Vitamins

For women whose dietary picture or whose laboratory test results indicate its appropriateness, multiple vitamins are prescribed with the addition at times of pyridoxine or magnesium. Those who support the use of pyridoxine suggest that it may be reduced in competitive inhibition by estrogen, may enhance estrogen clearance, and may augment biosynthesis of brain monoamines (Winston 1973; Reid and Yen 1983). In uncontrolled studies there have been suggestive beneficial effects of both pyridoxine and magnesium. However, it would seem important to emphasize that even such apparently innocuous treatments may not be free of side effects. In a recent study, the use of 2,000–6,000 mg of pyridoxine daily resulted in some signs of peripheral neuropathy (Schaumburg 1983), and the safety of even 400 mg daily has recently been questioned (Berger 1984). These symptoms gradually improved when the pyridoxine supplementation was discontinued. When used for premenstrual symptoms, both pyridoxine and magnesium have most commonly been prescribed in doses of 100–300 mg daily.

Progesterone

Natural progesterone given by rectal suspension or vaginal or rectal suppository has had numerous proponents both in the United States and elsewhere. It has been most popularized by the work of Katherina Dalton (1977) in England, who claimed to substantiate its benefits in large numbers of patients under a wide variety of circumstances. The theoretical rationale has rested on a relative progesterone deficiency or estrogen excess. To date, such hormonal imbalances have not been substantiated. It remains possible that the pharmacological doses used could have some unknown central nervous system effects that would relate to the amelioration of premenstrual symptoms; however, this needs further investigation. The two studies that have used progesterone in a double-blind design not only had other methodological problems but failed to substantiate the efficacy of progesterone treatment (Sampson 1979; Smith 1975). However, the treatment remains a widely utilized approach at the present time, and a number of clinicians believe that it has a useful role, at least for selected patients.

The usual starting dose of progesterone is 25–100 mg intramuscularly every other day or 200–400 mg daily by vaginal or rectal suppository from midcycle until the onset of menstruation; some physicians discontinue the progesterone one to two days prior to expected menstruation. If the dose does not control the symptoms, or if after a period of initial control the symptoms return, increasing amounts of progesterone have been applied, usually as much as 1,600 mg daily by suppository. To date, reported side effects have been relatively minor. Patients may experience sedation, dysphoria, and a worsening of depressive symptoms, especially if such symptoms have been a prominent component of the difficulty, and they may experience a worsening of vaginal candidiasis. Although no long-term difficulties have been substantiated, concern has been raised about possible long-term metabolic or neoplastic side effects in patients or subsequent generations. Because of the sedating qualities of progesterone, some have recommended it primarily for patients with symptoms of anxiety, irritability, or volatility. Similarly, because of side effects of depression, progesterone should be used with caution or in lower doses, if it is used at all, in women with primary symptoms of severe depression, especially if suicidal features are prominent (Schinfeld unpublished manuscript). It is not contraindicated in women with seizure disorders and, indeed, raises the threshold of seizures. Progesterone is not an effective contraceptive. Because of a possible very low incidence of fetal disorders, progesterone should not be started during a cycle in which unprotected intercourse has taken place, and women taking progesterone should be counseled to use appropriate contraception.

Medroxyprogesterone acetate tablets (Provera) and oral contraceptive steroids have also been used to treat premenstrual symptoms. Both regimens have the advantage of greater ease of administration and lesser cost compared with progesterone. As with progesterone, double-blind studies have not been performed that substantiate the efficacy of these treatments. In the studies that are available related to the use of medroxyprogesterone, improvement of symptoms, worsening of symptoms, and no differential effects from placebo have been reported. If medroxyprogesterone acetate tablets are used, the usual dose is 10–20 mg daily beginning on the 14th day of the cycle and being either discontinued at menstruation or tapered in the days prior to anticipated menstruation. As with medroxyprogesterone acetate, some women report dramatic improvement of premenstrual symptoms while taking oral contraceptive steroids and some report a worsening of symptoms; no study to date has substantiated the greater efficacy of oral contraceptive steroids compared with placebo. It is perhaps worth noting that isolated case reports have claimed an improvement of psychotic symptoms linked to the menstrual cycle when oral contraceptive steroids have been used as a component of the treatment regimen (Glick and Stewart 1980; Felthous et al. 1980). Oral contraceptives have proven effectiveness in dysmenorrhea. Therefore, for women younger than age 35, who require contraception, and especially for those in whom dysmenorrhea is a prominent symptom, oral contraceptives may be considered for therapy. When oral contraceptives are used, it is usually recommended that a progestagen-dominant contraceptive be employed, although this worsens symptoms in some groups.

Diuretics

Diuretics have been overutilized throughout the years for the treatment of premenstrual symptoms. It may be worth noting that the majority of women who report bloating do not have documented weight gain. For women with substantiated weight gain and edema, the first step should be a reduction in intake of salt and refined carbohydrates. When these measures are ineffective, some have claimed that pyridoxine will be efficacious. Spironolactone, an aldosterone antagonist and diuretic, has been claimed to be useful in the treatment of premenstrual symptoms (O'Brien et al. 1979). Most studies have not confirmed its efficacy. However, when menstrually related edema and weight gain are persistent and a trial of diuretics appears warranted, spironolactone, 25 mg four times per day, can be used during the period of active symptoms.

Bromocriptine

Because the possibility that prolactin abnormalities are related to premenstrual symptoms has been suggested, bromocriptine has been used as a treatment regimen (Anderson et al. 1979). To date, links to prolactin abnormalities remain tenuous, and benefits of bromocriptine also remain unsubstantiated. Bromocriptine is not an innocuous drug. Nausea is a frequent side effect, and patients may also experience such symptoms as headache, dizziness, or fatigue. Occasionally, hypotension may be noted. If there is hyperprolactinemia, further evaluation is warranted and bromocriptine treatment may be indicated. Furthermore, bromocriptine may be considered for the control of breast swelling and tenderness. The dose is 2.5 mg orally twice daily. Other medications that may be effective for the control of breast swelling and tenderness are spironolactone, 25 mg orally four times daily, and danazol, 200 mg orally twice daily (Reid and Yen 1983). Patients taking danazol sometimes report the development of acne, mild hirsutism, and decrease in breast size. Mild hypoestrogenic manifestations are sometimes seen. There are also reports of dizziness, muscle cramps, and gastrointestinal symptoms, usually of a mild nature. Patients receiving danazol should be advised to avoid conception during its use.

Antiprostaglandins

Antiprostaglandins clearly are efficacious in the treatment of dysmenorrhea. In general, however, they do not appear to have similar usefulness in the treatment of premenstrual symptoms although there are some suggestions that they may be of use in decreasing breast tenderness, abdominal bloating, ankle swelling, and edema. It is perhaps worth remembering that up until a decade ago, confusion around the etiology and treatment of dysmenorrhea was similar to that which now exists concerning many premenstrual symptoms. The documented usefulness of the antiprostaglandins for the treatment of dysmenorrhea may lend hope and presage development in the understanding and treatment of at least some categories of premenstrual syndromes.

Other Treatment Regimens

Other treatment regimens and research approaches are currently being used in a number of medical centers. One example is the use of a yeast-free diet combined with orally or vaginally administered mycostatin (Schinfeld unpublished manuscript). Another is the experimental elimination of ovarian cyclicity with a gonadotropin-releasing hormone agonist, with improvement of symptoms in a small number of cases (Muse et al. 1984). Careful studies of these and other approaches will be needed to assess their possible efficacy.

DISCUSSION

In this chapter we have attempted to consider approaches to evaluation and management of the premenstrual symptoms that clinicians encounter in practice. We have undertaken this task with the knowledge that theoretical underpinnings remain questionable and that clinical research has been confounded by methodological problems, with results for given approaches subsequently not being replicated. We recognize that future studies will provide important information about premenstrual symptoms, including evaluation and treatment strategies and the possible links between premenstrual syndromes and psychiatric symptoms. Yet, we are also aware that in the interim women in increasing numbers are requesting treatment for symptoms, that sensitive clinicians are independently linking symptoms to the menstrual cycle, and that clinicians are employing treatment regimens—even if unverified—for these symptoms.

We would stress the importance of a careful prospective evaluation prior to the initiation of any treatment. Significant numbers of patients will require no further treatment at the end of the period of evaluation. They may learn triggering factors, methods of decreasing pressures, and self-treatment techniques. Some feel more comfortable in living with their symptoms. Of those requiring treatment, a number of different patterns will be apparent.

A considerable number of women will have psychiatric symptoms but with patterns apparently unrelated to the menstrual cycle. We would emphasize that patients with psychiatric symptoms—even with a premenstrual component to their symptoms—should not be denied appropriate psychiatric treatment. Women whose symptoms appear related to the menstrual cycle warrant further assessment, and we recommend careful evaluation with emphasis on psychiatric, gynecological, medical, nutritional, and endocrinological components. Specific findings may emerge that explain symptoms that indicate specific treatment. We would emphasize that if clinicians are going to prescribe medications for premenstrual symptoms, they should recognize that the theoretical rationale and confirmatory data remain fragmentary and that approval by the Food and Drug Administration is lacking in most cases. We therefore advise clinicians to be cautious and use initially those approaches that appear to be pharmacologically safest, reserving other approaches for more refractory cases. We also encourage clinicians to look for side effects and provide careful follow-up to monitor treatment efficacy.

With this in mind, we have summarized some approaches that are currently being utilized for treatment of premenstrual symptoms. Overall approaches incorporate exercise; a well-balanced diet including decreased intake of refined sugars, coffee, tea, and chocolate; decreased alcohol consumption; and cutbacks in smoking. A number of treatment regimens include vitamins, progesterone—either natural progesterone, synthetic derivatives, or oral contraceptive steroids—diuretics, bromocriptine and other steroids, and antiprostaglandins. We have attempted to provide some logical guidelines on the basis of patient symptoms, clinical data, and research underpinnings. We hope that in future years newer conceptualizations and careful clinical studies will provide more coherent approaches to understanding, evaluating, and treating premenstrual symptoms.

REFERENCES

Andersen AN, Larsen JF: Bromocriptine in the treatment of the premenstrual syndrome. Drugs 17:383–388, 1979

Berger A, Schaumburg H: More on neuropathy from pyridoxine abuse (letter). N Engl J Med 311:936–987, 1984

Bertoli A, DePirro R, Fusco A, et al: Differences in insulin receptors between men and menstruating women in influence of sex hormones on insulin binding during the menstrual cycle. J Clin Endocrinol Metab 50:246–250, 1980

Carr DB, Bullen BA, Serinar GS, et al: Physical conditioning facilitates the exercise-induced secretion of beta-endorphin and beta-lipotropin in women. N Engl J Med 305:560–563, 1981

Dalton K: The Premenstrual Syndrome and Progesterone Therapy. London, William Heinemann Medical Books, 1977

Endicott J, Halbreich U, Schacht S, et al: Premenstrual changes and affective disorders. Psychosom Med 43:519–529, 1981

Felthous AR, Robinson DB, Conroy RW: Prevention of recurrent menstrual psychosis by an oral contraceptive. Am J Psychiatry 137:245–246, 1980

Frank RT: Hormonal causes of premenstrual tension. Archives of Neurological Psychiatry 26:1053–1057, 1931

Glick RD, Stewart D: A new drug treatment for premenstrual exacerbation of schizophrenia. Compr Psychiatry 21:281–287, 1980

Halbreich U, Endicott J: Classification of the premenstrual cycle, in Behavior and the Menstrual Cycle. Edited by Friedman R. New York, Marcel Dekker, 1984, pp 245–265

Muse K, Cetel NS, Futterman LA, et al: The premenstrual syndrome: Effects of "medical ovariectomy." N Engl J Med 311:1345–1349, 1984

Newmark NE, Penrey JK: Catamenial epilepsy. Epilepsia 21:281–300, 1980

O'Brien PM, Craven D, Selby D, et al: Treatment of premenstrual syndrome by spironolactone. Br J Obstet Gynecol 86:142–147, 1979

Reid RL, Yen SS: The premenstrual syndrome. Clin Obstet Gynecol 26:710–718, 1983

Rubinow DR, Roy-Byrne P: Premenstrual syndromes: Overview from a methodologic perspective. Am J Psychiatry 141:163–172, 1984

Sampson GA: Premenstrual syndrome: a double-blind controlled trial of progesterone and placebo. Br J Psychiatry 135:209–215, 1979

Schaumburg H, Kaplan J, Windeban K, et al: Sensory neuropathy from pyridoxine abuse. N Engl J Med 309:445–448, 1983

Schinfeld JS, Cronin L: Premenstrual syndrome. Unpublished manuscript

Smith SL: Mood and the menstrual cycle, in Topics in Psychoendocrinology. Edited by Sacher EJ. New York, Grune & Stratton, 1975, pp 19–58

Winston F: Oral contraceptives, pyridoxine, and depression. Am J Psychiatry 130:1217–1221, 1973

Chapter 5

Treatment of Premenstrual Syndrome in Psychiatric Practice

Ira D. Glick, M.D.

Chapter 5

Treatment of Premenstrual Syndrome in Psychiatric Practice

S ince this chapter deals with the treatment of premenstrual syndrome (PMS) in psychiatric practice, it will focus on severe PMS and exacerbation of psychiatric disorders rather than on mild or moderate PMS.

CLINICAL PROBLEMS

The clinical problems are somewhat different in severe PMS from those in premenstrual exacerbation of psychiatric disorders. In severe PMS, the clinician attempts to control an episodic, dysphoric state that produces relatively consistent (from cycle to cycle) mood and behavioral symptoms. In contrast, the problem in premenstrual exacerbation of psychiatric disorder is premenstrual reemergence of symptoms associated with the psychiatric disorder in question.

METHODOLOGICAL PROBLEMS

Symptoms may vary in intensity and duration from cycle to cycle in the same patient. Some cycles may be symptom free. The nature and severity of symptoms may vary over the life cycle. The syndromes appear to have multiple etiologies and subtypes.

The degree to which symptoms are dysfunctional is variable. One must therefore use goal-attainment scaling—individualized and rank ordered for each subject—as well as role and global scales. The severity of symptoms varies with the population studied (e.g., college students or patients referred from an obstetrical practice). There is a high rate of placebo response. Symptoms of PMS often overlap with those resulting from psychiatric illness. The severity of exogenous stress varies during the life of each patient. Judgment of outcome depends on who is assessing it (patient, significant other, or independent observer); and different outcomes are reported depending on whether the patient and significant other are interviewed together or apart and whether they are asked about their relationship or only about the PMS.

Many studies have inadequate controls and therefore pose serious problems in the interpretation of the data and the adequate comparison of one treatment with another. Usually it is necessary to compare an active drug with placebo or to compare two active drugs with placebo. To complicate matters, the response varies with the population. It appears necessary to have each patient serve as her own control, and most researchers indicate that the advantages of using a crossover design outweigh the disadvantages.

It is important to have a large enough study population so that the effects of other treatments for psychiatric illness may be disentangled from the treatment prescribed for PMS. And it is essential to obtain long-term cooperation and compliance from both the patient and her significant other.

RATIONALE FOR TREATMENT

Premenstrual Exacerbation of Psychiatric Disorders

Affective Disorders. The rationale for the use of lithium in the treatment of PMS has been that these syndromes are cyclic conditions that have many symptoms in common with affective disorders. It was therefore thought that PMS and affective disorders might share a similar etiologic thread, and the hope was that lithium would stabilize mood and behavior in PMSs as it does in some affective disorders.

Positive results have been achieved only in uncontrolled studies. Sletten and Gershon (1966) conducted an open study of eight patients, most of whom had agitated symptoms and all of whom improved. Fries (1969) reported improvement in two of five patients with PMS, and he believed that these two had an affective disorder. Deleon-Jones et al. (1982) reported the successful use of lithium to treat PMS in a woman with manic-depressive symptoms, a family history of premenstrual mania, and abnormal levels of 3-methoxy-4-hydroxyphenylglycol in urine.

However, double-blind, controlled studies have suggested that lithium is ineffective. These include the work of Mattson and van Shoultz (1974), who found lithium inferior to placebo, and the work of Singer et al. (1974), who compared lithium with placebo in a double-blind crossover-design study of 19 Chinese patients with mixed psychiatric diagnosis. Singer et al. found that patients improved on both regimens and that the differences between regimens were not significant.

Another approach to the treatment of PMS has been the use of tricyclic antidepressants and monoamine oxidase (MAO) inhibitors. Such drugs have been used alone or with synthetic progestins. The rationale is that premenstrual exacerbation of affective illness may share some etiologic mechanism with affective disorder; however, there have been no controlled studies of such treatment. I have used these drugs to treat recurrent, unipolar depressive disorders in a clinical setting and have obtained a decrease of premenstrual exacerbations in seven of eight patients. There are anecdotal reports claiming beneficial results of treatment of patients with MAO inhibitors, during the 10 days before the expected onset of menstruation, but most clinicians administer these drugs throughout the cycle. In those patients whose symptoms have been resistant to treatment, I have added medroxyprogesterone acetate (Provera) to the prescription and obtained a decrease in symptoms in about half of the patients. *Schizophrenic Disorders.* The rationale for treatment of exacerbation of schizophrenic disorders has been based on the observation that a small percentage of schizophrenic patients whose symptoms have been controlled by standard treatment (phenothiazines) develop severe premenstrual exacerbation of the same symptoms.

Treatment studies have all been uncontrolled. The first was the Blumberg and Billig (1942) study in which electroshock therapy or insulin coma treatments were combined with the administration of natural progesterone. (2 mg intramuscularly). The authors reported that all 12 patients had relief of symptoms. Wieczarek et al. (1969) used chlormadinone and mestranol to treat schizophrenic patients. Some of their patients improved and others had a worsening of symptoms. (The size of the study population was not specified.) Swanson et al. (1964) treated patients with Enovid (mestranol and chlormadinone). They reported that 21 of 26 patients improved; there was no change in four, and one relapsed.

Phenothiazines plus synthetic progestins or oral contraceptives plus lithium were used by Glick and Stewart (1980) in an uncontrolled study of three hospitalized patients with severe premenstrual exacerbation of schizophrenia. The symptoms of these patients could not be controlled with phenothiazines alone or with the addition of progestins or oral contraceptives; however, control was achieved in both the hospital and posthospital phases (one to two years) when lithium was added to the regimen. Felthous et al. (1980) used Ortho-Novum (mestranol and chlormadinone) to treat one patient who had highly resistant symptoms, and they reported a good response.

Berlin et al. (1982) used synthetic progesterone to treat a patient in early adolescence who had pubertal psychosis. The patient's symptoms ceased completely for more than one year. Cookson (1967) used clomiphene (an estrogen antagonist) in a patient with a recurrent psychosis and reported good results.

Borderline Personality Disorder.   Kane (1977) reported the results of treating one patient who had borderline personality disorder with an oral contraceptive, in this case, norethynodrel with mestronal. The patient's condition improved. Many clinicians have noted that a large percentage of female patients with borderline personality disorder also have PMS. There is a small subgroup of patients with borderline personality disorder who appear to have affective disorder as well. Therefore my approach to treating patients with borderline personality disorder has been to begin by determining whether affective disorder is also present. If it is, I prescribe either a tricyclic antidepressant or an MAO inhibitor. Depending on the nature of the clinical problem, I add a synthetic progestin or an oral contraceptive. The number of patients studied is too small to allow generalizable treatment recommendations.

Severe PMS Without Psychiatric Illness

Natural Progesterone.   Most reviewers of this literature begin by describing Dalton's experience (1977). She has anecdotally reported the results of more than 30 years of experience with a large but unspecified number of patients. She recommends natural rather than synthetic progesterone, administered intramuscularly, by suppository, or by subcutaneous implant. She has reported "very positive" results with "very few adverse effects" during a 10-year period.

There have been two controlled studies yielding negative results. Sampson (1979) found no significant differences when he compared natural progesterone (at doses of 200 mg and 400 mg twice daily administered by suppository or pessary) with placebo in a double-blind, crossover study. Smith (1976) administered progesterone intramuscularly and found no significant differences between results with progesterone and those with placebo.

It is of note that there are currently a growing number of clinics that specialize in the use of natural progesterone in the treatment of PMS. One clinic that uses progesterone in controlled conditions is that of Steege at Duke University. Steege administers the drug (100 mg twice daily) by suppository after establishing a baseline for symptoms. He has reported promising results in his first 15 patients; 13 improved and two dropped out (personal communication).

Synthetic Progesterones.   There have been three studies of dydrogesterone, a synthetic progesterone similar to the natural hormone. Taylor and James (1979), in an uncontrolled open trial, found that

70 percent of 50 patients with PMS (and lower than normal blood levels of progesterone) improved. The dose was 10 mg twice daily administered for the 14th through the 26th day of the reproductive cycle. Day (1979), in a single-blind, placebo-controlled study found improvement in 70 percent of patients receiving dydrogesterone compared with 40 percent in patients receiving placebo. Haspels (1981) in a double-blind study found a response rate of 75 percent in patients receiving dydrogesterone compared with 53 percent in those receiving placebo.

A pilot study performed by Glick and Goldfein in 1970 was later reported in an article by Glick and Bennett (1982). The study involved four subjects who had severe PMS characterized by a broad range of psychological and physiological symptoms without other psychiatric illness. They received Provera in oral doses of 10–20 mg for 10 days before the expected onset of menstruation. The subjects were studied over the course of 35 cycles, and the results indicated a mean improvement of 1.29 (on the three-point positive side of a seven-point global rating scale) above each subject's baseline levels (measured during two to four cycles).

Oral Contraceptives.   The data from three large controlled surveys (Herzberg and Coppen 1970; Kutner and Brown 1972; and Winston 1973) suggest that patients who have dysmenorrhea or severe premenstrual symptoms without significant psychiatric illness improved with administration of gestagen-dominant contraceptive pills. Oral contraceptives in which estrogen predominates appear to make the symptoms worse. However, a report of opposite findings by Lewis and Hoghughi (1969) highlights the confusion that exists in this area.

Lithium and Other Neurotropic Drugs.   Rosman (1969) used lithium to treat eight women, 31–41 years of age, who had premenstrual tension. They had previously not responded to psychotropic or diuretic drugs. The women received lithium at a dose of 300 mg three times daily for 10–14 days. Rosman reported that "in all cases response was good, with no side effects in seven, but one patient stopped because of severe itching."

Perhaps of more importance, Steiner et al. (1980) studied 15 patients with severe PMS in a double-blind study of lithium vs. placebo that extended through three cycles. Only five patients improved, and of these only three agreed to stay on the study regimen after the study ended. The authors concluded that lithium was ineffective.

A number of clinicians have used lithium to treat patients in whom the symptoms of severe PMS seemed to resemble those of agitated depression. In such patients there appears to be a positive response. This kind of clinical intuition remains to be documented in controlled studies. Pyridoxine and bromocriptine (a dopamine agonist) have also been used. Results for both drugs are inconclusive. Other newer approaches include the use of atropine (an anticholinergic agent that is also a dopamine blocker) based on the rationale that there is dopaminergic overactivity. It is still too early to evaluate such approaches.

Psychotherapy.   In my experience, external stress is not a consistent trigger for PMS. Thus it is not surprising that individual psychotherapy prescribed without medication does not consistently improve target symptoms. I believe that in some cases martial therapy is indicated to deal with interpersonal effects of the syndromes and to increase compliance with pharmacologic treatment.

SUMMARY AND RECOMMENDATIONS

One way to view the problem of PMS is to consider a model that includes both premenstrual exacerbation of preexisting psychiatric illness and PMS without concomitant psychiatric illness. It is important to recognize that PMS may vary in intensity, may exist independently of psychiatric illness, and may predispose the patient (or lead directly) to a depressive disorder. The pathophysiologic mechanisms of PMS and psychiatric illness are probably separate but may share some overlapping features.

My primary recommendation is a call for controlled studies. I believe that the time is right for prospective, comparative treatment interventions like those used during the 1960s in the development of pharmacologic treatments for psychiatric disorders. In that case the strategy was to delineate syndromes on the basis of responses to promising drugs, and a placebo control was sometimes used.

My methodological recommendations for treatment studies include the following: Studies should probably be collaborative because of the problems in obtaining sufficiently large numbers of subjects. Furthermore, in view of the large individual variation in symptoms, drug-free baseline data must be obtained during at least three cycles. Baseline data are also needed to compare posttreatment symptom levels with pretreatment levels. The studies must be double blind and should be placebo controlled.

The samples should be delineated clearly with the use of standardized diagnostic criteria, such as those in the DSM-III, and standard diagnostic instruments, including the schedule for affective disorders and schizophrenia, lifetime (SADS-L) or the Structured Clinical Interview for DSM-III (SCIDS). Populations should be defined by age, socioeconomic class, and nature of referral source. Length of the study must be at least six months, preferably 24 months, because of the fluctuations of symptoms in each cycle and because external life events vary from cycle to cycle. Treatment must be standardized and specific. Drugs must be administered in adequate doses during adequate lengths of time. (The importance of the latter requirement has been noted in earlier generations of psychopharmacologic studies.)

Measures of outcome must be taken from the vantage point of patient, significant other, and independent assessor. The areas considered should include symptoms, work function, and social function as well as global outcome which, I believe, is the most important. Independent assessment is crucial in this area. Ratings should be made daily, monthly, and biannually. I believe that there is value in retrospective evaluation of a particular time period. This rating is useful simply because it provides a different vantage point, that is, the view of hindsight. The severity of symptoms must be rated, and I find it useful to construct a narrative describing the course of each patient's symptoms.

I would like to emphasize that at present no drug has proven efficacy in the treatment of PMS. I believe that we are at an early stage in this work and that an acceptable strategy is to conduct controlled, high-quality clinical studies that compare various promising treatments.

REFERENCES

Berlin FS, Bergey GK, Money J: Periodic psychosis of puberty: a case report. Am J Psychiatry 139:119–120, 1982

Blumberg A, Billig O: Hormonal influence upon "puerperal psychosis" and neurotic conditions. Psychiatr Q 16:454–462, 1942

Cookson BA: Clinical note on the possible use of clomiphene citrate in recurrent psychosis. Can J Psychiatry 11:271–274, 1967

Dalton K: The Premenstrual Syndrome and Progesterone Therapy. London, William Heinemann Medical Books, 1977

Day JB: Clinical trials in the premenstrual syndrome. Curr Med Res Opin 6:40–45, 1979

Deleon-Jones FA, Val E, Herts C: MHPG excretion and lithium treatment during premenstrual tension syndrome: a case report. Am J Psychiatry 139:850–852, 1982

Felthous AR, Robinson DB, Conroy RW: Prevention of recurrent menstrual psychosis by an oral contraceptive. Am J Psychiatry 137:245–246, 1980

Fries H: Experience with lithium carbonate treatment at a psychiatric department in the period 1964–67. Acta Psychiatr Scand. [Suppl] 207:41–43, 1969

Glick ID, Bennett SE: Oral contraceptives and the menstrual cycle, in Behavior and the Menstrual Cycle. Edited by Friedman RC. New York, Marcel Dekker, 1982, pp 345–365

Glick ID, Stewart D: A new drug treatment for premenstrual exacerbation of schizophrenia. Compr Psychiatry 21:281–287, 1980

Haspels AA: A double-blind, placebo-controlled, multicentre study of the efficacy of dydrogesterone (Duphaston), in The Premenstrual Syndrome. Edited by van Keep PA. Lancaster, England, MTP Press, 1981

Herzberg B, Coppen A: Changes in psychological symptoms in women taking oral contraceptives. Br J Psychiatry 116:161–164, 1970

Kane FJ: Iatrogenic depression in women, in Phenomenology and Treatment of Depression. Edited by Fann WE, Karcan I, Polorny A. New York, Spectrum, 1977

Kutner SJ, Brown WL: Types of oral contraceptives, depression and premenstrual symptoms. J Nerv Ment Dis 155:153–162, 1972

Lewis A, Hoghughi M: An evaluation of depression as a side effect of oral contraceptives. Br J Psychiatry 115:697–701, 1969

Mattson B, von Schoultz B: A comparison between lithium, placebo and a diuretic in premenstrual tension. Acta Psychiatr Scand [Suppl] 255:75–83, 1974

Rosman C: Discussion (with data on lithium administration against premenstrual tension). Acta Psychiatr Scand 207:89, 1969

Sampson GA: A double-blind controlled trial of progesterone and placebo. Br J Psychiatry 135:209–215, 1979

Singer K, Cheng R, Schou M: A controlled evaluation of lithium in the premenstrual tension syndrome. Br J Psychiatry 124:50–51, 1974

Sletten JW, Gershon S: The premenstrual syndrome: a discussion of its pathophysiology and treatment with lithium ion. Compr Psychiatry 7:197–206, 1966

Smith SL: The menstrual cycle and mood disturbances. Clin Obstet Gynecol 19:391–397, 1976

Steiner M, Haskett RF, Osmun JN, et al: Treatment of premenstrual tension with lithium carbonate. Acta Psychiatr Scand 61:96–102, 1980

Swanson D, Barron A, Floren A, et al: The use of norethynodrel in psychotic females. Am J Psychiatry 120:1101–1103, 1964

Taylor RW, James CE: The clinician's view of patients with premenstrual syndrome. Curr Med Res Opin 6:46–51, 1979

Wieczarek V, Bock R, Kluge H: Use of ovulation inhibitors in female epileptics and psychiatric patients. MMW 111:254–259, 1969

Winston F: Oral contraceptives, pyridoxine, and depression. Am J Psychiatry 130:1217–1221, 1973

Chapter 6

Cognitive Approaches to Understanding and Treating Premenstrual Depressions

Jean A. Hamilton, M.D.
Sheryle W. Alagna, Ph.D.
Kathey Sharpe, M.A.

Chapter 6

Cognitive Approaches to Understanding and Treating Premenstrual Depressions

B oth research and clinical data indicate that among a vulnerable subgroup of women, affective and other symptoms consistent with various subtypes of depression occur episodically, with a timing that appears linked to the premenstrual phase (Endicott et al. 1981). Although Beck and Rush (1979) and Weingartner et al. (1981) have described in detail the types of cognitive alterations that are characteristic in affective disorders, the cognitive component of depressive changes linked to the menstrual cycle has received much less attention.

The significance of the menstrual cycle is highlighted by some women's premenstrual self-reports which are heavily focused on changes consistent with cognitive theories of depression. These reports include a premenstrual loss of interest in activities that usually provide positive reinforcement, an increased sense of vulnerability or helplessness, and a decreased belief that external events are controllable or that one can control one's own behavior.

On the other hand, reviews of the empirical literature on effects of the menstrual cycle reveal that women's self-perceptions of a premenstrual impairment in performance are in most instances not confirmed by objective measures (Sommer 1983). Women typically do not perform any differently during the premenstrual phase than during other portions of the menstrual cycle, although their reported differences suggest that they may think differently about themselves or about events that occur (Parlee 1982). For this reason, we have become interested in possible alterations in self-perceptions that may occur for some women premenstrually. Just as distorted or maladaptive self-assessments may be evidence for cognitive-perceptual disturbances in depression (Beck and Rush 1979) or in anorexia (Slade and Russell 1973), we believe that the discrepancy between self-reports and observer ratings (Gotlieb and Robinson 1982) or actual performance measures (Thayer 1971) may be important in understanding depressive mood changes that occur premenstrually.

Moreover, part of the gender difference in the prevalence of depression may come from the tendency of women to encode, recall, or consolidate depression-related experiences into their self-image somewhat differently from men. In particular some women may preferentially retain and use information congruent with culturally stereotyped and negative images or expectations of women. For example, even before puberty and the onset of menstruation, females in our society are more likely to overgeneralize performance failures, attributing deficits to a lack of ability—which is uncontrollable—rather than to lack of effort (Dweck and Reppucci 1973). This difference has been linked to increased negative affect and lowered self-esteem (Frieze 1975). In this chapter we will consider whether some women may find this tendency exacerbated premenstrually, thereby increasing their risk for the onset of mood disturbances; this hypothesis can be seen, in part, as a reinterpretation of the work of Benedeck and Rubenstein (1939), who first investigated possible menstrually related effects on psychodynamic processes and on self-esteem.

In order to explore cognitive approaches to understanding and treating premenstrual depressions, we will examine possible menstrual cycle effects in several models of cognitive functioning. The finding that gonadal hormones, such as progesterone, play a role in state-dependent learning may provide a biological model for the investigation of cycle-phase effects on cognition. Because of possible cyclic effects of these hormones on the putative biological substrates of learned helplessness models, we will explore an attributional approach to conceptualizing menstrual cycle–linked depressive cognitions. We will present clinical parallels to these models and discuss treatment implications. We believe that cognitive approaches, although in need of further elaboration and testing, are useful as guides to understanding and treating premenstrual depressive mood changes. Because some of the findings to be reported are counterintuitive, we have provided a summary (Table 1) in order to help orient the reader.

POSSIBLE MENSTRUAL CYCLE–LINKED EFFECTS ON COGNITION

Neisser has defined cognition as "all of the processes by which the sensory input is transformed, reduced, elaborated, stored, recovered, and used" (1967, 4). In a review of menstrual effects on cognition, Sommer (1983) concluded that "among the general population of women, menstrual cycle variables do not interfere with cognitive abilities—abilities of thinking, problem-solving, learning and memory, making judgments, and other related activities." Although there is some evidence for small menstrual cycle–related changes in sensory acuity and sensitivity and in motor activity, the data on these sensory-motor effects are mixed. Parlee (1983) has documented a complicated pattern of both enhanced and diminished performance effects by cycle phase depending upon the type of task and sensory modality involved. These observations suggest that for most women effects of the menstrual cycle on primary intellectual abilities are minimal.

The possibility remains that a subgroup of women experience alterations in cognitive functioning that are linked to the cycle phase and that may accompany and/or exacerbate premenstrual depressive symptoms. For example, some women appear to be more susceptible to conditioning procedures premenstrually (Asso and Beech 1975), and these conditioned responses may be more resistant to extinction than are those acquired at other times in the cycle (Vila and Beech 1977). The responsivity to repeated external stimuli may also be altered premenstrually, with preliminary evidence suggesting more rapid habituation in this cycle phase (Friedman and Meares 1979). However, because simple performance deficit models have been shown to be inadequate, we will explore more complex accounts of possible effects of menstrual cycle phase on conditioning, habituation, and other indexes of information processing.

State-Dependent Learning by Phase of the Menstrual Cycle

It is well established that recall is enhanced in situations—or in neurochemically defined states—that are congruent with those in which encoding occurred. We are all familiar, for example, with the experience of greater ease in recalling song titles, and their words, as a record is being played, as opposed to in a noncued, free-recall situation. Another example of situation-dependent cognition is the reactivation of drug-craving or drug-related ideas that may occur in ex-addicts who visit environments in which they formerly used drugs. In addition, mood-state–dependent learning and recall have been demonstrated clinically. For example, depressed patients retrieve previously learned information less completely when remembering occurs in a mood state that is different from the one experienced at the time of storage (Weingartner et al. 1977).

The fact that both drugs and hormones have been shown to produce state-dependent effects on learning and memory (Weingartner and Murphy 1977) has been viewed by Hamilton et al. (1983c) as suggesting that the hormonal milieu of the premenstrual phase may partially define a neurochemical or emotional state that affects learning and recall, perhaps by activating previously conditioned cogni-

Table 1. Cognitive Findings and Treatment Implications

Approaches to Cognitive Functioning	Preliminary Findings	Treatment Implications
Psychodynamic	• Ovarian cycle affects self-image and ego strength (Benedek and Rubenstein 1939).	• To listen for cycle-phase effects on self-image and on self-perceptions.
Discrepancies in self-reports	• The discrepancy between concurrent and retrospective self-reports of menstrual cycle related symptoms suggests a bias in information processing (Parlee 1982).	• To facilitate self-awareness (e.g., a diary method).
	• Globally reported premenstrual symptoms are associated with negatively biased self-perceptions of performance (Hamilton and Alagna, this chapter).	• To encourage women not to discount premenstrual cognitions automatically, but to view those changes as meaningful data about the self that can be placed in the wider context of experiences in other phases of the cycle.
Learned helplessness	• The biological basis of these effects in animal studies may be affected by menstrual cycle–related physiological changes in women (Maier 1983; Hamilton et al. 1983).	
	• Attributional models are pertinent to menstrually related symptoms (Koeske and Koeske 1975; Ruble and Brooks-Gunn 1979).	• To address the internalization of stereotypes that devalue women (because these may be triggered by the menstrual cycle, an obvious biological reminder of being female).

Approaches to Cognitive Functioning	Preliminary Findings	Treatment Implications
	• Premenstrual women as compared with intermenstrual women may feel more responsible for their interactions with others (Alagna and Hamilton, in press).	• To help women to avoid internal, global, and stable attributions.
	• The uncontrollability dimension may be especially salient for some women's menstrual cycle–related experiences.	
State-dependent learning	• Hormones play a role in state-dependent learning (Weingartner and Murphy 1977). There may be menstrual cycle–related effects on learning and recall (Hamilton et al. 1983).	• To address state-dependent discontinuities in information processing.
	• Anecdotal clinical reports suggest menstrual cycle–related effects in information processing (Hamilton and Alagna, this chapter).	
Cognitive theories of depression	• Beck's conceptualization of maladaptive thinking may be pertinent to premenstrual mood changes.	• To address the logical errors of over-generalization (e.g., the devaluation of women), selective abstraction (focusing on the premenstrual phase as the sole determination of negative moods), personalization (sense of being unique in these experiences), and dichotomous thinking and magnification.

tions or self-perceptions. That is, the impact of experiences or information processed premenstrually may be differentially reinforced by cyclic activation or recall in cycle-phase congruent states. A preliminary study by Weingartner and colleagues (unpublished data) is consistent with effects of the menstrual cycle on state-dependent learning.

ATTRIBUTIONAL MODELS OF CYCLE-PHASE EFFECTS ON LEARNING

Socioendocrinology and the Argument Against Biological Reductionism

We do not believe that hormone or drug-induced neurochemical changes directly determine our experiences. Instead, it is well known that drug-induced effects are shaped by expectations and cognitive labeling (Schachter and Singer 1962) and by the environment (cf. McQuire 1982), including social dominance hierarchies. The strongest argument against biological reductionism in cognitive research comes from the recognition of reciprocal effects of the environment (both social and physical) and neuroendocrine functioning. As we have discussed elsewhere (Hamilton et al. 1984), a variety of contextual stimuli including social contacts with other females (McClintock 1983; Hrdy 1981, especially chapter 6), can influence characteristics of the menstrual cycle. Even relatively acute stress can affect circulating levels of gonadal steroids in males (Rose 1980) and may also interfere with the patterns of LH secretion necessary for ovulation.

Learned Helplessness, Depression, and the Menstrual Cycle

Cognitive theories generally emphasize the importance of positive rewards, controllability (Abramson et al. 1978), and adaptive patterns of thinking (Beck and Rush 1979) in the regulation of mood. The learned helplessness theory of depression specifically emphasizes the perceived uncontrollability of rewarding and punishing events. The attributional reformulation of the learned helplessness model links depression to the types of causal attributions that people make to account for a lack of control in their lives (Abramson et al. 1978). The attributions made in a given situation reflect both a stable tendency of the individual—based in part on culturally prescribed stereotypes and beliefs—and the information currently available. Depression is thought to result from self-perceptions of a failure to control situations in accordance with one's values or goals. In particular, internal, global, and stable attributions for such failures give rise to depression.

Koeske and Koeske (1975) applied an attributional model to menstrual cycle research. According to their conceptualization, beliefs about menstruation and gender-related self-concepts are linked to physical and emotional symptoms through a chain of causal attributions. In a social cognition analysis, Ruble and Brooks-Gunn (1979) also discuss how beliefs about characteristic features of a cycle phase— as opposed to actual cycle-phase effects—help to shape symptomatology. Chernovetz et al. (1979) reported that women who were more accepting of culturally defined, gender-related expectations experienced more severe symptoms of menstrual discomfort.

Following up on these attributional models, Alagna and Hamilton (in press) compared women in different portions of the menstrual cycle with each other, and with men, in their responses to a social interaction stimulus (a videotape depicting a female nurse interacting with a hospitalized patient). In addition to differences along both affective and cognitive dimensions, premenstrual women made significantly greater attributions of responsibility (control) to the behavior of the dominant person (nurse) toward the person with a subordinate role (patient) than did intermenstrual women. This finding is consistent with the hypothesis that some women may be inclined to feel more responsible for the nature and quality of their interactions with others when they are in the premenstrual phase. Their internal attributions of responsibility—in the face of their actual lack of complete control—could give rise to heightened feelings of helplessness, guilt, or depression in negative situations.

Moreover, menstruation itself may be associated with the experience of uncontrollability, particularly for those women who are not able to predict its onset. In fact, because of normal irregularity, many women are occasionally unprepared for their period. Even when the onset is predictable, other characteristics, such as the severity of cramping or the intensity of the flow, may not be. For example, an unexpectedly heavy flow may contribute to feelings of "uncontrollability." A transient, heightened sense of vulnerability or helplessness may be realistic in the case of such accidental events as staining one's clothes, and these events may be experienced as both somewhat traumatic and as evidence of a failure to make adequate preparations. According to this perspective, irregular cycles can be expected to be associated with greater menstrually related distress; preliminary data from our clinical study show a trend toward support of this hypothesis ($r = .34$, $df = 16$, $p = .088$). However, one can also argue that having premenstrual symptomatology may actually help some women to predict the onset of their period, thereby decreasing the experienced uncontrollability, so that we would expect the interrelationships to be complex (cf. Chernovetz et al. 1979).

In order to apply a learned helplessness model to the menstrual cycle, it is necessary to show that cycle phase–linked learning gives rise to the expectation that future outcomes are independent of one's current responses (helplessness). The variability of the menstrual cycle experienced by some women may contribute to this sense of response-outcome independence. Just as learned helplessness has been applied to the understanding of traumatic life events, (Peterson and Seligman 1983), we believe that efforts should be made to clarify its possible application to premenstrual conditionability. Since the Attributional Style Questionnaire (Peterson et al. 1982) is not yet well validated, we have begun a study in which high- and low-symptom groups are tested premenstrually and postmenstrually with tasks in which the level of control is experimentally varied. We anticipate that tasks in which the level of control is low will have more influence on self-perception of affect in premenstrual women than in postmenstrual women.

Reports of Premenstrual Distress and Self-Perceptions of Cognitive Performance

Further evidence for a link between premenstrual symptoms and cognition comes from a study of self-perceptions. Using an approach that is detailed elsewhere (Hamilton et al. in press), we compared self-ratings of cognitive functioning with actual behavior on the continuous performance test (CPT), which is a measure of sustained attention. A subgroup of 26 subjects responded to requests for follow-up testing as part of a larger community college–based survey ($N = 97$) on the menstrual cycle.

All subjects were screened for a premenstrually related symptomatology with the use of the Menstrual Distress Questionnaire (Moos 1968), which reflects global, one-time, retrospective reports. The 12 high-symptom subjects had a mean intermenstrual baseline score of 75 (± 8) with a mean symptomatic increase of 79 percent reported premenstrually. The nine low-symptom subjects had a similar mean baseline score of 81 (± 13) but showed virtually no change premenstrually (range, 13 percent to 21 percent). A third comparison group of five subjects had a mean premenstrual increase of about 25 percent but will not be further discussed here. Preliminary analyses were performed for three of the five CPT summary scores: the total number correct, errors of commission (an index of impulsivity), and errors of omission (an index of distractability). Self-ratings included items on concentration, boredom, attentional involvement, distractability, and the wish to be doing something else.

Data from the 17 subjects in the high- and low-symptom groups who were tested in the first half of their cycles are reported here, since the groups tested premenstrually are very small, presumably because of self-selection. Our findings primarily reflect differences for groups defined by global self-reports, rather than direct effects of cycle phase itself.

The high-symptom ($N = 10$) and low-symptom ($N = 7$) groups that were tested intermenstrually did not differ on any CPT measure except for errors of commission. The self-identified high-symptom group made significantly fewer errors of commission (mean $\pm$ SEM, 3.4 ± 0.82) compared with the low-symptom group (5.4 ± 0.60). This suggests that women who incorporate recollections of premenstrual distress into their stable self-image actually show less impulsivity as assessed by intermenstrual errors of commission on the CPT. For the high-symptom group, there was a significant discrepancy between errors of commission and reports of concentration, and the discrepancy was such that reports of poor concentration were actually associated with better performance ($r = -.67$, $df = 9$, $p \leqslant .05$), whereas the low-symptom group showed the expected positive relationship ($r = .54$, $df = 6$, $p \geqslant .10$) ($t = 2.26$, $p < .05$).

Despite the fact that global, retrospective self-reports of premenstrual symptomatology are not necessarily confirmed by concurrent measures (Hamilton et al. 1984), it appears that there are differences between these self-identified groups in self-perceptions. A biological difference that has been reported for these globally defined subgroups (Hamilton et al. 1983) may be an additional source of external validation for these global groups. In a separate study, a high-premenstrual-symptom group ($n = 3$) had an average score of 150 on the Moos test (B-scale), and a low-symptom group ($n = 3$) had an average score of 65. Daily 24-hour urine samples were collected across two cycles, and levels of 6-hydroxymelatonin, a metabolite of the pineal hormone melatonin, were measured by gas chromatographic spectrometry. The high-symptom group had a mean level of 9.2 ± 1.5 μg/day and the low-symptom group had a mean of 15.8 ± 2.4 μg/day, a 1.7-fold greater level that was relatively stable across the month. Perhaps these differences reflect menstrually related effects on the information about the self that becomes incorporated into one's self-image or consolidated into personality. We believe that, taken together with other work on menstrual cycle–related self-perceptions, these preliminary findings support further exploration of possible menstrual effects on processing information about the self.

THE BIOLOGICAL SUBSTRATE OF MENSTRUAL CYCLE-RELATED EFFECTS ON COGNITION

Certain neurons in sensory projection areas as well as in other neural circuits are sensitive to gonadal steroids. Learned behaviors such as maze performance also appear to be mediated by groups of developing neurons that are sensitive to steroids (cf. McEwen 1981). Moreover, gonadal and adrenal steroids are known to affect neuroregulatory systems that help to modulate sensory or cognitive processing (Rubinow et al. 1984).

Opiod pathways, which are thought to play a role in sensory processing hierarchies (Lewis et al. 1981), represent a specific example. The same prohormone that gives rise to β-endorphin also gives rise to adrenocorticotropic hormone (ACTH) (Cooper and Martin 1982), which stimulates adrenal cortisol, thereby helping to mediate responsivity to stress. In monkeys, the level of β-endorphin in hypophyseal portal blood depends on adequate circulating levels of gonadal steroids. As summarized in a brief review by Hamilton et al. (1983a), the levels of β-endorphin in monkeys rise premenstrually and fall to undetectable levels with the onset of menstruation. However, because of difficulties in obtaining reliable and specific measures of ACTH, preliminary reports of human menstrual variation must be viewed with caution.

In animals, chronic intermittent stress seems to elicit learned helplessness and a sensory analgesia that is partly mediated by opiates (Miczek et al. 1982). The uncontrollability that is characteristic of the stressor is thought to be crucial in determining both the occurrence of the analgesia reaction and its opiod nature (Maier 1983). In view of steroid and cycle-related effects on endogenous opiates, there exists a strong rationale for investigating possible estrous effects on the determinants of learned helplessness in animals.

Clinical parallels may include the decreased perception of pain by depressed patients as well as by women in the premenstrual phase (Parlee 1983). An ACTH fragment (4-10) appears to have a slight effect on attentional performance in women, although possible menstrual cycle effects have not been investigated (Veith et al. 1978). Along with dexamethasone and progesterone, ACTH is known to elicit state-dependent learning (Weingartner and Murphy 1977). Differences in cortisol hypersecretion have been correlated with differences in performance on the Halstead Category Test in depressed patients compared with normal controls; however, age was a confounding variable, and a partial correlation—which might have better delineated these effects—was not performed (Rubinow et al. 1984).

Clinical Parallels and Treatment Implications

State-Dependent Learning. One of us (J.H.) has seen several patients in psychotherapy who have expressed heightened emotional turmoil and vulnerability to interpersonal rejection during therapy sessions preceding menstruation but who claimed virtual amnesia about these concerns in sessions the following week. The discontinuity is not observed in these patients except for the premenstrual-to-intermenstrual phase of the cycle. Premenstrually, however, these women may refer to the previously "forgotten" sessions when they had struggled with issues such as hostile dependency. Hence, there is anecdotal clinical evidence that is pertinent to models of state-dependent learning and recall in the menstrual cycle.

Just as individuals may express certain concerns almost exclusively in drug-induced states, some women appear to split off and isolate certain affects to the premenstrual phase. These women often conceptualize conflict-laden feelings or behaviors as occurring only in alien phases of the cycle when they are "not themselves." Just as alcoholic state-dependent processing is described in the saying "in vino veritas" (in wine there is truth), the issues expressed by these women premenstrually may in fact be central rather than peripheral to their difficulties, despite claims to the contrary. One of the goals with these patients is to break down the state-dependent discontinuities in their processing of information about themselves and their environment. When the memory and recognition of affects are facilitated across all phases of the menstrual cycle, the patients will begin to create a more integrated and autonomous self-image that can span both time-of-the-month and interpersonal conflict.

Learned Helplessness. Despite mixed findings in the literature, women's unequal social role (Carmen et al. 1981) and stereotyped expectations of passivity almost undoubtedly contribute to a kind of learned helplessness. The therapist must be sensitive to the effects of economic inequality, subordinate group status, vulnerability to victimization, situational and social role stressors, and the internalization of culturally prescribed stereotypes that devalue women. To help women avoid the possible heightened impact of negative self-perceptions and expectations premenstrually, the therapist should help patients to construct external, unstable, and specific—rather than global—explanations for their negative "uncontrollable" experiences. That is, an important aspect of cognitive therapy is informational: women are told that they need not see all premenstrual symptoms as evidence of "craziness," that there must be some reason if they are angry and that their anger need not be uncontrollable, that being a woman does not mean that one must be passive and dependent, and that their concerns are shared by many women.

In particular, more adaptive ways of viewing the cycle should be encouraged. The Menstrual Attitude Questionnaire (Brooks-Gunn and Ruble 1980) includes several positive assessments of the menstrual cycle that may be useful approaches to cognitive restructuring. For example, some women report feeling more in touch with nature or with their bodies premenstrually. Some women may find it useful to know that 10 percent to 15 percent of women report positive changes premenstrually and that Olympic gold medals have been won around the time of menstruation (Walsh et al. 1981). Another cognitive restructuring technique is to remind the patient that other stressors may provoke similar symptomatology. For example, although the menstrual cycle is an obvious biological reminder of being female, the realization that a minor academic examination or a flat tire can elicit degrees of irritability and helplessness similar to those experienced premenstrually may decrease the inappropriate global attribution of all premenstrual symptomatology to something about womanhood.

Because anticipatory planning can enhance a woman's sense of control, the therapist should assist her in efforts to predict and better manage upcoming stresses and to be aware that the premenstrual phase may be a time of altered responsivity. One positive approach is to help women view premenstrual changes as an opportunity to attend to, experience, and learn about aspects of themselves that may be less salient or not evident at all other times in the cycle. Another strategy is to encourage women to view premenstrual changes as meaningful data about the self that can be placed into the wider context of her experiences in other phases of the cycle. Self-monitoring techniques can assist a patient in assessing her own experience across the menstrual cycle. An additional strategy is to have women record their life experiences several times a day, using a daily diary or some other technique for repeated real-time sampling (Hamilton et al. 1984). This will develop a more precise, accurate, and objective conceptualization of life experience, which in itself may enhance a woman's sense of control. The act of self-observation implies that one's experiences deserve to be taken seriously and helps reinforce the view that compensatory strategies for self-control can be developed.

Beck's analysis of maladaptive thinking patterns can be applied to certain premenstrual depressive complaints. Some women appear to believe that constant "stability" is the norm and that transient mood fluctuations are totally unacceptable and are signs of weakness and incompetence. A more realistic appraisal is that we all have ups and downs and that some of these may reflect physiological rhythmicity. We have already touched on the logical errors of overgeneralization (devaluation of women), and personalization (a sense of being unique in these experiences). Selective abstraction can be seen in focusing on the premenstrual phase as the sole determinant of negative moods or behavior, conceptualizing an entire experience on the basis of this one detail. Dichotomous thinking and magnification may sometimes be evidenced in describing one's life in bipolar terms such as that occurring premenstrually ("I'm totally a failure") versus all other times ("I'm a great success"). In fact, some women are helped by clarifying their tendency to overlook changes that occur throughout the rest of their menstrual cycle.

The general therapeutic approach that we are advocating is essentially metacognitive: helping each women to refine her awareness of her own mental processes. All of the relationships proposed here are in need of further elaboration and testing. Ultimately, we hope to gain a better understanding of the ways in which psychological, biochemical, and social factors influence and interact with processes of the menstrual cycle in the regulation of mood. It appears that expectations and self-perceptions play an important role in shaping the outcome of whatever physiological changes may be occurring premenstrually. We believe that examples such as these demonstrate the usefulness of cognitive approaches to understanding and treating premenstrual depressive mood changes.

REFERENCES

Abramson, LY, Seligman MEP, Teasdale JD: Learned helplessness in humans: critique and reformulation. J Abnorm Psychol 89:49–74, 1978

Alagna SW, Hamilton JA: Social stimulus perception and self-evaluation: effects of menstrual cycle phase. Psychology of Women Quarterly (in press)

Asso DK, Beech HR: Susceptibility to the acquisition of a conditioned response in relation to the menstrual cycle. J Psychosom Res 19:337–344, 1975

Beck AT, Rush AJ: Cognitive approaches to depression and suicide, in Cognitive Defects in the Development of Mental Illness. Edited by Serban G. New York, Brunner/Mazel, 1979

Benedek T, Rubenstein BB: Correlations between ovarian activity and psychodynamic processes [in two parts]. Psychosom Med 1:245–270, 461–485, 1939

Brooks-Gunn J, Ruble DN: The Menstrual Attitude Questionnaire. Psychosom Med 42:503–512, 1980

Carmen (Hilberman) E, Russo NF, Miller JB: Inequality and women's mental health: an overview. Am J Psychiatry 138:1319–1330, 1981

Chernovetz ME, Jones WH, Hansson RO: Predictability, attentional focus, sex role orientation, and menstrual-related stress. Psychosom Med 41:383–391, 1979

Cooper PE, Martin JB: Neuroendocrinology and brain peptides. TINS June:186–189, 1982

Dweck CS, Reppucci ND: Learned helplessness and reinforcement in children. J Pers Soc Psychol 25:109–116, 1973

Endicott J, Halbreich U, Schacht S, et al: Premenstrual changes and affective disorders. Psychosom Med 43:519–530, 1981

Friedman J, Meares RA: The menstrual cycle and habituation. Psychosom Med 41:369–381, 1979

Frieze IH: Women's expectations for and causal attributions of success and failure, in Women and Achievement, Social and Motivational Analyses. Edited by Mednick MTS, Tangri SS, Hoffman LW. New York, John Wiley & Sons, 1975, pp 158–171

Gotlieb I, Robinson LA: Responses to depressed individuals: discrepancies between self-report and observer-rated behavior. J Abnorm Psychol 91:231–240, 1982

Hamilton JA, Alagna SW, Pinkel S: Gender differences in antidepressant and activating drug effects on self-perceptions. J Affective Disord (in press)

Hamilton JA, Aloi J, Mucciardi B, et al: Human plasma β-endorphin through the menstrual cycle. Psychopharmacol Bull 19:586–587, 1983a

Hamilton JA, Aloi J, Mucciardi B, et al: A neuroendocrine evaluation of premenstrual syndrome. Presented at the Annual Meeting of the American Psychosomatic Society, New York, March 1983b

Hamilton JA, Parry BL, Alagna S, et al: Premenstrual mood changes: a guide to evaluation and treatment. Psychiatric Annals 14:426–435, 1984

Hamilton JA, Sharpe K, Mucciardi B, et al: Menstrual changes: a model for research and therapy. Presented at the 136th Annual Meeting of the American Psychiatric Association, New York, May 1983c

Hrdy SB: The Women That Never Evolved. Cambridge, Harvard University Press, 1981

Koeske R, Koeske G: An attributional approach to moods and the menstrual cycle. J Pers Soc Psychol 3:473–478, 1975

Lewis ME, Mishkin M, Bragin E, et al: Opiate receptor gradients in monkey cerebral cortex: correspondence with sensory processing hierarchies. Science 211:1166, 1981

Maier SF: Learned helplessness, depression, analgesia and opiates. Presented at the Annual Meeting of the American College of Neuropharmacology, San Juan, Puerto Rico, December 1983

McClintock MK: The behavioral endocrinology of rodents: a functional analysis. Bioscience 33:573–577, 1983

McEwen BS: Neural gonadal steroid actions. Science 211:1303–1311, 1981

McQuire MT: Sociopharmacology. Annu Rev Pharmacol Toxicol 22:643–661, 1982

Miczek KA, Thompson ML, Schuster L: Opioid-like analgesia in defeated mice. Science 215:1520–1523, 1982

Moos RH: The development of a menstrual distress questionnaire. Psychosom Med 30:853–867, 1968

Neisser U: Cognitive psychology. New York, Appleton-Century-Crofts, 1967

Parlee MB: Changes in moods and activation levels during the menstrual cycle in experimentally naive subjects. Psychology of Women Quarterly 7:119–131, 1982

Parlee MB: Menstrual rhythms in sensory processes: a review of fluctuations in vision, olfaction, audition, taste, and touch. Psychol Bull 93:539–548, 1983

Peterson C, Seligman MEP: Learned helplessness and victimization. Journal of Social Issues 2:103–116, 1983

Peterson C, Semmel A, von Baeyer C, et al: The attributional style questionnaire. Cognitive Therapy and Research 6:287–299, 1982

Rose RM: Endocrine responses to stressful psychological events. Psychiatr Clin North Am 3:251–276, 1980

Rubinow DR, Post RM, Savand R, et al: Cortisol hypersecretion and cognitive impairment in depression. Arch Gen Psychiatry 41:279–283, 1984

Ruble DR, Brooks-Gunn J: Menstrual symptoms: a social cognition analysis. J Behav Med 2:171–194, 1979

Schachter S, Singer JE: Cognitive, social, and psychological determinants of emotional state. Psychol Rev 69:379–399, 1962

Slade PD, Russell GFM: Awareness of body dimensions in anorexia nervosa: cross-sectional and longitudinal studies. Psychol Medicine 3:188–199, 1973

Sommer B: How does menstruation affect cognitive competence and psychophysiological response. Women and Health 8:53–88, 1983

Thayer RE: Personality and discrepancies between verbal reports and physiological measures of private emotional experiences. J Pers 89:57-69, 1971

Veith JL, Sandman CA, George JM, et al: Effects of MSH/ACTH 4-10 on memory, attention, and endogenous hormone levels in women. Physiol Behav 20:43–50, 1978

Vila J, Beech HR: Vulnerability and conditioning in relation to the human menstrual cycle. Br J Soc Psychol 16:69–75, 1977

Walsh RN, Budtz-Olsen I, Leader C, et al: The menstrual cycle, personality, and academic performance. Arch Gen Psychiatry 38:219–221, 1981

Weingartner H, Miller H, Murphy DL: Mood-state-dependent retrieval of verbal associations. J Abnorm Psychol 86:276–284, 1977

Weingartner H, Murphy DL: Brain states and memory: state-dependent storage and retrieval of information. Psychopharmacol Bull 13:66–67, 1977

Weingartner H, Cohen RM, Murphy DL, et al: Cognitive processes in depression. Arch Gen Psychiatry 38:42–47, 1981

Chapter 7

Research Techniques Used to Study Premenstrual Syndrome

Barbara L. Parry, M.D.
Norman E. Rosenthal, M.D.
Thomas A. Wehr, M.D.

Chapter 7

Research Techniques Used to Study Premenstrual Syndrome

Certain features of the premenstrual syndrome (PMS) make it especially suitable for scientific investigation. There is an inherent link between the premenstrual affective changes and a specific physiologic process, the menstrual cycle. In contrast, most other forms of affective illness have not been linked to any known physiologic process. Thus, the menstrual cycle, an identified physiologic trigger for PMS, can be considered a proximate, though not an ultimate, cause of PMS and can serve as a point of departure for generating hypotheses about its pathogenesis.

Another advantage of studying PMS is that mood and behavioral changes are recurrent and predictable and can be studied prospectively and longitudinally. In contrast to many other psychiatric disorders in which the precipitating and alleviating influences are not easily identified and may be mediated through different mechanisms, in PMS the causative and curative mechanisms are both entrained to the menstrual cycle. The fact that a common physiologic process is involved in remission and relapse helps to focus investigation into the pathophysiology of PMS.

In spite of the apparent methodological advantages of studying PMS, research in this area has been handicapped by a lack of precision in diagnosis and in measurements (Rubinow 1984a). Furthermore, many studies have been carried out with no specific testable hypothesis in mind. In this chapter we discuss approaches to clinical assessment, to problems of methodology, and to hypothesis development. From these approaches, new techniques are being derived to study PMS.

LONGITUDINAL APPROACH TO DIAGNOSIS AND MEASUREMENTS

Course of the Illness and Diagnosis

To improve clinical PMS research, recent work has focused on diagnostic procedures. Improved diagnosis helps to decrease heterogeneity of the sample population and to obtain more consistent findings. To diagnose PMS it is necessary to identify and observe longitudinally the types of symptoms that follow a characteristic course and achieve a certain intensity.

Prospective ratings across several menstrual cycles are necessary in order to establish the temporal relationship of symptoms to phases of the menstrual cycle. The inadequacy of retrospective reports is demonstrated by the fact that only 20 percent to 50 percent of them are actually confirmed by prospective observations (Endicott and Halbreich 1982). This discrepancy itself deserves investigation.

Since many women experience some physical or psychological changes premenstrually, it is important to establish criteria for severity that can separate pathologic from physiologic premenstrual changes. Unfortunately, the use of longitudinal self-ratings to establish a diagnosis is complicated by interindividual differences in self-observation and symptom reporting. This interindividual variation in sensitivity makes it difficult to determine a threshold for change that will include pathologic cases and exclude normal women. Though some investigators (Rubinow 1984b) recommend the use of daily ratings to establish a diagnosis, we are finding that such frequent measurements may be too sensitive to day-to-day changes unrelated to the menstrual cycle. No reliable method for removing random error or accounting for irrelevant cyclic variations has been developed in PMS research.

At the present state of knowledge, global self-ratings, such as analogue mood scales, should be complemented by multi-item mood inventories and observer rating scales, such as the Hamilton Rating Scale for Depression, done at least weekly. A National Institute of Mental Health conference recommended that when such scales are used, a diagnosis of PMS should be made only when mean symptom intensity changes at least 30 percent in the premenstrual period (six days before menses) compared with the intermenstrual period (days 5–10 of the cycle). Furthermore, items to be measured should be specific for PMS symptoms. Factors such as irritability, hostility, or fatigue need to be added to standardized depression rating scales in order to make them valid for PMS.

The symptoms of PMS vary considerably among individuals. It is unclear whether diverse symptoms arise from a single disease process or multiple ones. To decrease sample heterogeneity further, recent work has focused on delineating diagnostic subgroups. For example, Halbreich et al. (1983) have identified subtypes of premenstrual symptoms and are attempting to determine their frequency and reliability. Individual differences in expressions of symptomatology may be influenced by psychological, situational, or sociocultural factors or may arise from different biologic substrates. Only by careful documentation of the clinical, biologic, and genetic characteristics of identified subgroups can it be determined whether they represent distinct syndromes or are different manifestations of the same illness.

Variance Due to Timing of Measurements

Many studies have used single time points to determine measurements. Unfortunately this sampling strategy does not take into account daily and monthly rhythmic variations and does not lend itself to understanding how biologic processes change. For a 28-day cycle, spans between successive measurements should certainly be no more than seven days in order to delineate changes associated with the menstrual cycle. In studying cyclic phenomena, the phase of the cycle in which measurements are obtained must be determined. In PMS research, differing or inadequate methods for measuring menstrual cycle phase or accounting for variation in total cycle length may be responsible for inconsistency of findings. The same cycle day may reflect different menstrual cycle phases in women with different cycle lengths. Thus, reliance on external time markers, rather than internal ones, can increase variability due to menstrual phase differences among individuals. To standardize menstrual phase definitions it is desirable to relate menstrual day to menstrual stage with cytologic, hormonal, or body temperature measurements. To further reduce variability due to phase differences arising from biologic rhythms, month of the year should be reported, since there may be circannual changes in menstrual rhythms (Reinberg and Smolensky 1974).

Variation due to circadian (near 24-hour) rhythms is often quite large and may be greater than that associated with the menstrual cycle or PMS. For example, prolactin, which has been a focus of investigation and theory in PMS, exhibits plasma levels that are many times higher during sleep at night than during wakefulness in the daytime (Sassin et al. 1972). If 24-hour profiles of variables of interest were obtained at weekly intervals throughout the menstrual cycle, they would provide information about the contribution of circadian variation to measurements and about possible alterations in the circadian system in PMS.

HYPOTHESIS DEVELOPMENT

Many biologic investigations of PMS have measured a wide variety of variables with no specific hypothesis in mind. A problem with this lack of focus is that some of the multitude of biologic variables measured will prove statistically significant by chance alone unless conservative statistical methods are used.

As more descriptive research is done, specific hypotheses about the pathogenesis of PMS need to be developed. Furthermore, these hypotheses need to be tested by systematic investigation using pharmacologic or other experimental perturbations. For example, prolactin has been implicated in the pathogenesis of PMS (Carroll and Steiner 1978). To test this hypothesis, we have examined prolactin responses to thyrotropin-releasing hormone infusions in women with PMS and are investigating behavioral changes in women with idiopathic hyperprolactinemia to determine whether the symptoms of hyperprolactinemia resemble those of PMS.

There are several sources from which hypotheses about the pathogenesis of PMS can be derived. One approach has been to base hypotheses about causes of PMS on observations of patterns of covariation between specified variables (e.g., hormone levels and mood, or mood state and phase of menstrual cycle). This type of research provides a useful description of the illness but has limitations. From a description of variables that covary across the menstrual cycle one cannot infer a causal relationship. Furthermore, it is difficult to distinguish between normal menstrual cycle variations unrelated to PMS and variations (normal or abnormal) that cause or participate in PMS. For example, many neuroregulatory processes may vary across the menstrual cycle but may not be involved in PMS.

Attempts to determine whether an excess or a deficiency of a particular hormone occurs premenstrually in PMS have not been successful and therefore have not led to specific hypotheses. This lack of success may be due to the wide range of inter- and intraindividual variation in hormone levels in normal women. Surprisingly, investigators have interpreted changes in variables associated with PMS as abnormal without defining normal menstrual cycle variations. Of course, control populations are needed in PMS studies in order to define the degree of fluctuation that constitutes pathology.

Another approach has been to infer causes of premenstrual changes from treatment responses. For example, progesterone deficiency has been postulated to be responsible for PMS because some women's symptoms improve with progesterone treatment. However, effective treatment may act through a mechanism that is independent of the one responsible for PMS. Another pitfall of inferring pathogenesis from treatment response is the high rate of placebo response (about 60 percent) in PMS (Day 1979).

In interpreting results of their studies, investigators frequently have not taken into account spontaneous remissions (regression to the mean), nonspecific therapeutic effects of the treatment situation, or the effect of expectations on treatment outcome. These problems highlight the need for double-blind, placebo-controlled, crossover designs in treatment studies.

Another strategy for hypothesis development has been to import hypotheses and methods from affective disorder research to PMS studies. The relation of PMS to affective disorders remains to be determined. The roles of catecholamine and neuroendocrine levels, circadian rhythm, and sleep disturbances, which have been implicated in the pathogenesis of affective disorders, have not been systematically investigated in PMS. For example, changing levels of 3-methoxy-4-hydroxyphenylglycol, homovanillic acid, 5-hydroxy-indoleacetic acid, and monoamine oxidase that were hypothesized to reflect alterations in monoamine neurotransmitter function and to be involved in pathologic mood states, are now being specifically measured in PMS studies. In some theories of PMS, changing levels of estrogen and progesterone have been thought to alter monoamine neurotransmitter function (Rausch et al. 1982) and thereby to alter mood. There is support for this theory based on animal work showing the effects of gonadal steroids on neurotransmitter metabolism (McEwen and Parson 1982). An initial approach to testing this hypothesis would be to measure and examine patterns of covariations of monoamines and gonadal steroids across the menstrual cycle in normal and symptomatic women and then systematically challenge relevant systems with pharmacologic or other experimental perturbations. Unfortunately, changes in monoamine neurotransmitter function have not been proven to be related specifically to affective disorders or to be linked directly to their pathogenesis. Neuroendocrine abnormalities found in affective disorders (abnormal results in the dexamethasone suppression test and the thyrotropin-releasing-hormone test) are now being sought in PMS patients. Given the cyclic nature of PMS, and the probable interaction of daily and menstrual rhythms, the role of the circadian system in the pathogenesis of PMS deserves further investigation.

Sleep disturbance is a frequent feature of PMS. A project in progress is designed to determine whether sleep EEG patterns exhibit cyclic changes in PMS and, as in affective disorders, whether manipulations of the sleep-wake cycle, such as total or partial sleep deprivation, can ameliorate symptoms. A therapeutic response to sleep deprivation would be relevant to existing pathogenetic theories that attribute PMS symptoms to prolactin, inasmuch as sleep deprivation lowers prolactin levels (Parker et al. 1980; Sassin et al. 1973). Sleep deprivation has not proven to be clinically useful in the treatment of depression because of the tendency of symptoms to recur after recovery sleep. However, given that the duration of symptoms in PMS is sometimes limited to a few days, repeated total or partial sleep deprivation may prove practical and clinically effective.

It may also be useful to study the relationship between PMS and affective syndromes. For example, it is interesting that two forms of affective disorder also predominate in women and have predictable cyclic recurrences: rapid-cycling manic depressive illness and seasonal affective disorder (SAD) (Dunner 1979; Kukopolous et al. 1980; Rosenthal et al. 1984a).

Rapid-cycling manic depressive illness, defined as four or more affective episodes per year (Dunner 1979), predominates in women. Frequently these women have thyroid and reproductive hormone abnormalities (Cowdry et al. 1983), which may predispose them to the development of this illness, and thyroid hormone has been used to treat the disorder (Stancer 1982). Thyroid function and thyroid treatment have not been extensively investigated in PMS.

Seasonal affective disorder is characterized by depressions with atypical features (hyperphagia, hypersomnia, lethargy) that occur annually in the winter. Most of these patients respond to high-intensity (2,500 lux) light treatments which artificially extend the daily photoperiod (Rosenthal 1984a).

It has been hypothesized that bright light acts therapeutically by suppressing melatonin, a hormone released from the pineal gland (Rosenthal 1984b). A large proportion of the SAD population (70 percent) have mood disturbances premenstrually, which are also alleviated by light treatment. In an effort to explore the possible relationship between PMS and SAD, our group identified a patient who had PMS only in the winter and was virtually asymptomatic during the summer. We hypothesized that bright light might also be effective in this patient with seasonal PMS and might act by suppressing melatonin, a hormone that is centrally involved in the regulation of seasonal reproductive cycles in animals. We found that light was an effective treatment for PMS symptoms and that its therapeutic effect could be blocked by the simultaneous administration of melatonin. Propranolol, a β-blocker, which inhibits the synthesis of melatonin, had a therapeutic effect similar to light.

With these strategies we have provided some experimental support for the hypothesis that melatonin is involved in the pathogenesis of seasonal PMS. Induction of PMS symptoms by melatonin administered during the summer months would lend further support to the hypothesis that seasonally changing levels of melatonin are triggering PMS in this patient. Results obtained from single case studies cannot be generalized to other patients with PMS. Such research, however, serves a useful function as a pilot study or as an opportunity to carry out labor-intensive or expensive longitudinal investigations of multiple variables simultaneously. Such research does not replace but rather complements and inspires simpler investigations of groups of subjects. In future studies it would be important to attempt to relate PMS to other reproductive-related depressions (those depressions occurring in association with oral contraceptives, termination of pregnancy, pregnancy, the postpartum period, and menopause). The relationship of reproductive hormones to affective changes may be a common pathophysiologic feature of these disorders and PMS. Longitudinal studies need to be done to determine whether one such reproductive-related affective episode sensitizes a woman to the subsequent development of another type of reproductive-related depression. For example, there is some evidence that postpartum "blues" may be more severe in women with PMS and that mania and depression that occur postpartum are likely to recur premenstrually (Stein 1982). Research techniques designed to examine specific clinical and biologic links of PMS to periodic affective disorders in women could provide a basis for understanding the relationship of reproductive physiology to depression.

SUMMARY

Episodes of PMS are linked to a specific phase of the menstrual cycle, and they recur predictably. These features make PMS particularly suitable for prospective longitudinal approaches to scientific investigation. In PMS research, diagnosis and biobehavioral measurements must be related to the course and phases of the menstrual cycle to reduce inter- and intrasubject variability. Investigators need to be guided by specific hypotheses that can be tested experimentally. This approach may yield insights into causative mechanisms involved in the illness and may increase understanding of other forms of cyclic affective disorder in women.

REFERENCES

Carroll BJ, Steiner M: The psychobiology of premenstrual dysphoria: the role of prolactin. Psychoneuroendocrinology 3:171–180, 1978

Cowdry RW, Wehr TA, Zis AP, et al: Thyroid abnormalities associated with rapid cycling bipolar illness. Arch Gen Psychiatry 40:414–420, 1983

Day JB: Clinical trials in premenstrual syndrome. Current Medical Research and Opinion 6(Suppl 5):40–45, 1979

Dunner DL: Rapid cycling bipolar manic depressive illness. Psychiatr Clin North Am 2:461–467, 1979

Endicott J, Halbreich U: Retrospective reports of premenstrual changes: factors affecting confirmation by daily ratings. Psychopharmacol Bull 18:109–112, 1982

Halbreich U, Endicott J, Nee J: Premenstrual depressive changes. Arch Gen Psychiatry 40:535–542, 1983

Kukopolous A, Reginaldi D, Laddomada P, et al: Course of the manic depressive cycle and changes caused by treatments. Pharmacopsychiatry 13:156–167, 1980

McEwen BS, Parson B: Gonadal steroid action on the brain: neurochemistry and neuropharmacology. Annu Rev Pharmacol Toxicol 22:555–598, 1982

Parker DC, Rossman LG, Kripke DF, et al: Endocrine rhythms across sleep-wake cycles in normal young men under basal state conditions, in Physiology in Sleep. Edited by Orem J, Barnes CD. New York, Academic Press, 1980

Rausch JL, Janowsky DS, Risch SC, et al: Hormonal and neurotransmitter hypotheses of premenstrual tension. Psychopharmacol Bull 18:26–34, 1982

Reinberg A, Smolensky H: Circatrigintan secondary rhythms related to hormonal changes in the menstrual cycle: general considerations, in Biorhythms and Human Reproduction. Edited by Ferin M, Halberg F, Richard R, et al. New York, John Wiley & Sons, 1974

Rosenthal NE, Sack DA, Gillin JC, et al: Seasonal affective disorder: a description of the syndrome and preliminary findings with light therapy. Arch Gen Psychiatry 41:72–80, 1984a

Rosenthal NE, Sack DA, James SP: Seasonal affective disorder and phototherapy. Presented at the Annual Meeting of the New York Academy of Sciences, November 1984b

Rubinow DR, Roy-Byrne P: Premenstrual syndromes: overview from a methodological perspective. Am J Psychiatry 141:163–172, 1984a

Rubinow DR, Roy-Byrne P, Hoban CM, et al: Prospective assessment of menstrually related mood disorders. Am J Psychiatry 141:684–686, 1984b

Sassin JF, Frantz AG, Weitzman ED, et al: Human prolactin: 24-hour pattern with increased release during sleep. Science 177:1205–1207, 1972

Sassin JF, Frantz AG, Kapen S, et al: The nocturnal rise of human prolactin is dependent on sleep. J Clin Endocrinol Metab 37:436–440, 1973

Stancer HC, Persad E: Treatment of intractable rapid cycling manic depressive disorder with levothyroxine. Arch Gen Psychiatry 39:311–312, 1982

Stein G: The maternity blues, in Motherhood and Mental Illness. Edited by Brockington IF, Kumar R. London Academic Press, 1982